NUTRITION FOR A HEALTHY MOUTH

SECOND EDITION

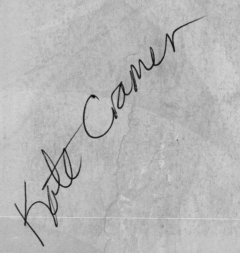

NUTRITION FOR A HEALTHY MOUTH

SECOND EDITION

Rebecca Sroda

**ASSOCIATE DEAN OF ALLIED HEALTH
AND DENTAL EDUCATION**

South Florida Community College
Avon Park, Florida

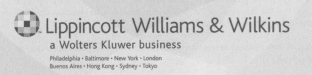 Lippincott Williams & Wilkins
a Wolters Kluwer business

Philadelphia · Baltimore · New York · London
Buenos Aires · Hong Kong · Sydney · Tokyo

Acquisitions Editor: John Goucher
Managing Editor: Meredith Brittain
Marketing Manager: Allison Noplock
Production Manager: Tom Gibbons
Design Coordinator: Stephen Druding
Production Services: Laserwords Private Limited, Chennai, India

351 West Camden Street
Baltimore, Maryland 21201-2436 USA

530 Walnut Street
Philadelphia, PA 19106 USA
LWW.com

Printed in China

Library of Congress Cataloging-in-Publication Data

Sroda, Rebecca.
Nutrition for a healthy mouth / Rebecca Sroda.—2nd ed.
    p. ; cm.
  Includes bibliographical references and index.
  ISBN-13: 978-0-7817-9825-9 (alk. paper)
  ISBN-10: 0-7817-9825-6 (alk. paper)
  1. Nutrition and dental health. 2. Mouth–Diseases–Nutritional aspects. 3. Dental assistants. 4. Nutrition. I. Title.
  [DNLM: 1. Mouth Diseases—diet therapy. 2. Dental Assistants. 3. Nutritional Physiological Phenomena. 4. Oral Hygiene. WU
    113.7 S774n 2009]
    RK281.S67 2009
    617.6′01—dc22

                                                                                          2008052225

Care has been taken to confirm the accuracy of the information presented and to describe generally accepted practices. However, the authors, editors, and publisher are not responsible for errors or omissions or for any consequences from application of the information in this book and make no warranty, expressed or implied, with respect to the currency, completeness, or accuracy of the contents of the publication. Application of this information in a particular situation remains the professional responsibility of the practitioner.

The authors, editors, and publisher have exerted every effort to ensure that drug selection and dosage set forth in this text are in accordance with current recommendations and practice at the time of publication. However, in view of ongoing research, changes in government regulations, and the constant flow of information relating to drug therapy and drug reactions, the reader is urged to check the package insert for each drug for any change in indications and dosage and for added warnings and precautions. This is particularly important when the recommended agent is a new or infrequently employed drug.

Some drugs and medical devices presented in this publication have Food and Drug Administration (FDA) clearance for limited use in restricted research settings. It is the responsibility of health care providers to ascertain the FDA status of each drug or device planned for use in their clinical practice.

To purchase additional copies of this book, call our customer service department at (800) 638-3030 or fax orders to (301) 223-2320. International customers should call (301) 223-2300.

Visit Lippincott Williams & Wilkins on the Internet: at LWW.com. Lippincott Williams & Wilkins customer service representatives are available from 8:30 AM to 6 PM, EST.

10 9 8 7 6 5 4 3 2 1

To Jill Nield-Gehrig,
friend and mentor extraordinaire

FOREWORD

The second edition of *Nutrition for a Healthy Mouth* sets the new standard for dental nutrition textbooks. This book truly makes the topic of dental nutrition interesting and easy to learn. For educators, *Nutrition for a Healthy Mouth, second edition* provides all the elements for a comprehensive dental nutrition course.

New learning aids in the second edition include key terms, objectives, and a glossary. Food for Thought boxes assist students in applying nutrition concepts to patient care. Nutrients at a Glance charts provide easy access to important information. Perhaps the most valuable feature of this new edition, created for the reader, is materials to individualize a PowerPoint presentation for the patient being counseled. Templates and instructions make this task simple and will greatly enhance counseling sessions.

For educators, the second edition of *Nutrition for a Healthy Mouth* provides a wealth of teaching resources. The Instructor Resource website includes new comprehensive PowerPoint presentations for each chapter, a 250-question test bank, and suggestions for using content in the classroom. The Instructor Resource website guides the course instructor in ways to enhance student application of nutritional concepts including role-plays, blank counseling forms, and two complete case studies.

The second edition of *Nutrition for a Healthy Mouth* includes valuable new content including information that reflects the changing eating patterns and nutrition challenges in modern North American society: portion distortion, consumption norms, the glycemic index and ketosis, and obesity. A discussion of popular diets—Atkins, South Beach, Zone, Weight Watchers—prepares students to offer dental nutritional counseling to patients who are following one of these diets. Information on reading nutritional labels assists students in acquiring this important life skill and prepares them to educate patients on the importance of reading labels. New content on counseling special patient groups—such as older adults, cancer patients, the homeless, substance abusers, and the developmentally disabled—is especially helpful when faced with their particular eating challenges.

Nutrition for a Healthy Mouth, second edition marks the end of the "dry as dust" dental nutritional textbook—it is a wonderful, engaging textbook for dental hygiene and dental assisting students. This book excels in presenting the concepts of dental nutrition in a manner that facilitates the application of dental nutritional counseling in a clinical setting.

Jill S. Nield-Gehrig, RDH, MA
Dean Emeritus, Division of Allied Health
and Public Service Education
Asheville-Buncombe Technical Community College

Nutrition for a Healthy Mouth, second edition is a textbook for dental hygiene and dental assisting students and a reference for practicing clinicians.

- Dental hygiene students, who take but one nutrition course, can use the text as all encompassing for both a general and dental-related study of nutrition.
- Dental hygiene students who take a general nutrition course before enrolling in the program will find this book useful for a quick review of biochemistry before embarking on an in-depth study of nutritional counseling suggestions and techniques.
- Dental assisting students whose curriculum allows for only a few weeks of nutritional study may select appropriate topics to cover information required in their curriculum.
- Practicing clinicians will find the 24 hour, 3-day and 7-day diet diaries helpful in assessing the patient's diet for nutritional adequacy and increased risk of oral disease (see Chapter 16). If change is needed, most chapters contain a "Counseling Patients" section that includes suggestions that will prove useful when redesigning a patient's eating habits.

Nutrition is a complex, constantly evolving subject. It is the author's hope that this new edition proves to be an excellent learning tool for dental hygiene and dental assisting students, as well as for practicing clinicians.

ORGANIZATIONAL PHILOSOPHY

Reading the first chapter sets the stage for counseling patients in the 21st century, reminding the reader that our eating practices and lifestyle are very different from previous generations. After this introductory chapter (Part I), there are two main sections of the book:

- Part II (Chapters 2 to 8) highlights biochemistry of the six major nutrients plus herbs. *Nutrients at a Glance* charts in these chapters contain common categories of information to help the reader organize and compare details. This section of the book provides a solid science foundation on the chemical

nature of nutrients and provides insight for making healthy food choices for a long and healthy life.
- Parts III, IV, V, and VI (Chapters 9 to 17) relate the biochemical nature of nutrients to oral disease, healthy food choices, dental nutritional counseling, and the psychosocial aspects of food and eating. Successfully counseling patients on the relationship between diet and oral disease is a learned process that requires a blend of the clinician's knowledge, good communication skills, and appropriate nutritional intake and dietary forms.

CHAPTER FEATURES AND NEW CONTENT

Each chapter of *Nutrition for a Healthy Mouth, second edition* contains the following features:

- *Key terms*—new to this edition—highlight important concepts the student must understand. Terms are listed at the beginning of the chapter and defined in a glossary.
- *Objectives*—new to this edition—set out the learning goals for each chapter.
- *Food for Thought* boxes—a new feature of this edition——highlight chapter facts and facilitate application of topics to the real-life setting. The information recapped in the *Food for Thought* boxes is easy to read and designed to reinforce the reader's understanding of chapter content.
- *Putting This into Practice* sections at the end of each chapter provide activities that allow the reader to "work" with information and give the subject a practical application. These sections serve as a vehicle for the reader to critically think about topics covered. Completing the activities and solving the problems assists the reader in assimilating key chapter content.
- *Web Resources* at the end of each chapter lists websites that can be book-marked in "favorites" for a quick check of facts. The author made every effort to include the most current research and theories; however, in some aspects writing about nutrition is like trying to catch butterflies with a bottomless net. One study may recommend eliminating as much fat from the diet as possible and another may encourage inclusion of certain "good" fats. One day you may read a report that butter is bad for your arteries and the next day read that it is *ok* in moderation. In a discipline such as nutrition, where the body of knowledge is constantly expanding, the clinician must constantly update his or her knowledge to assure that the best advice is being given to patients. The best way to stay current is to make a habit of visiting reliable nutrition-related websites, frequently.

- As previously mentioned, *Nutrients at a Glance* charts in Part II contain common categories of information to help the reader organize and compare details of major nutrients and herbs.

For this edition, the last chapter, "Special Nutritional Needs" (Chapter 17), was expanded to include new content on patients with cancer, HIV, who are homeless, or substance abusers. When given the opportunity to provide nutritional counseling for patients in special groups, the clinician must think outside the box. Just as we are taught that oral hygiene instructions must be individualized to suit the patient's needs, so must nutritional counseling efforts.

ADDITIONAL RESOURCES

Nutrition for a Healthy Mouth, second edition includes additional resources for both instructors and students that are available on the book's companion website at thePoint.lww.com/ Sroda2e.

Instructors

Approved adopting instructors will be given access to the following additional resources:

- Brownstone test generator
- Image bank containing figures, tables, Putting This into Practice boxes, and Counseling Patients lists
- PowerPoint presentations, including dietary calculation questions for use with interactive clicker technology
- Nutritional counseling forms, including case studies and blank forms for practical use
- Role-playing exercises

Students

Students who have purchased *Nutrition for a Healthy Mouth, second edition* have access to the following additional resources:

- Template for individualized counseling sessions with their clients
- Nutritional counseling forms and blank forms for practical use

In addition, purchasers of the text can access the searchable Full Text Online by going to the *Nutrition for a Healthy Mouth, second edition* website at http://thePoint.lww.com/Sroda2e. See the inside front cover of this text for more details, including the passcode you will need to gain access to the website.

CONTENTS

PART V
FOOD FOR GROWTH   249

PART VI
NUTRITIONAL COUNSELING   281

PART I

INTRODUCTION

CHAPTER 1

EATING 101

OBJECTIVES

Upon completion of this chapter, the reader should be able to:

1 Discuss the evolution of the food industry from 20th to 21st century
2 Consider 21st century trends when recommending healthy food choices for patients
3 Describe the difference between a food habit and food craving
4 Explain the relationship between proportion distortion and obesity
5 List diseases associated with unhealthy food choice habits
6 Name two different types of food cravings
7 Outline the journey of food during the digestive process
8 Discuss current and future trends in nutrition

KEY TERMS

Consumption Norm	Food Habit	Nutrition
Enzyme	Gastrointestinal Tract	Peristalsis
Food Craving	Nutrients	Proportion Distortion

How we feed and nourish ourselves and children is not the same experience as it was for our parents. Meal planning, preparation, and eating are very different in the 21st century than in the last, which makes our lives unique compared with that of previous generations. We have mutated the concept of family mealtime with the help of food processing plants, the fast food industry, and mass marketing concepts.[1,2] The emergence of ready-made and frozen dinners has increased the popularity of a massive food processing industry, which gives us a new way to "restaurant" and allows "cooks" to broaden their horizons. Mom is no longer in the kitchen baking cookies when the kids come home from school, and dinner is not always on the table when the "bread winner" returns home after a long, hard day at work. Families find themselves without a chief cook in the kitchen and consuming 65% of all meals in their cars. When we order a meal from a restaurant, four out of five times we are sitting in a car.[3,4] We stop and pick up breakfast on our way to work, grab a quick bite for lunch, and stop for fast food in the evening before getting to our final destination. Thanks to the food industry's 20th century influence, most of us can drink breakfast from a bottle, eat lunch out of a box, and dinner from a carton. Gone are the days when the whole family gathers around a well-set table, at the same time everyday, partaking of a meal that took 2 hours to prepare. That kind of elegant dining is reserved only for special occasions.

When we view MyPyramid, we have to consider it through the eyes of someone living in the 21st century: we have to remember that all those pictures of delicious looking fruits and vegetables are not in our yards, ready to be picked off the vine or tree, that bread is not baking in the oven, and that we do not eat "three square meals" a day. Most of us are very busy people so we embrace the convenience of ready-made and fast food choices.

In your daily practice, consider the trends of the 21st century as you guide patients to choose food wisely. Understanding current trends enables individuals to make mindful choices that are both healthy for the body and accomodate current lifestyles. The following are current lifestyle standards and should be acknowledged when advising patients on making healthy food choices[2,4–6]:

- We have a tendency to eat on the run.
- People are surpassing the life expectancy age, creating a vast aging population with their own unique set of health problems.
- Adult obesity has doubled in the last 20 years—food portions are four times what they were.
- Although we are more aware of the benefits of daily exercise we remain sedentary, spending more time in front of the TV or computer.
- More hours per day are spent at work, putting more stress on the body.

FOOD CHOICES AND NUTRIENT NEEDS

Nutrition is what we choose to eat and put into our bodies, and the food we select contains **nutrients**—chemical substances that provide the body with energy and everything else it needs to function. Ninety-six percent of human body mass is composed of the elements oxygen, carbon, hydrogen, and nitrogen. These elements also make up the six major nutrients found in food, making the saying "you are what you eat" really ring true. We need to eat every day to provide the body with a steady supply of fuel, which is created by digestion and absorption of six major nutrients: carbohydrates, proteins, lipids, water, vitamins, and minerals. Often, our bodies, in their own subtle way, will let us know which foods to choose to get the necessary nutrients. When we are dehydrated, we thirst for water (hydrogen and oxygen); when our activity level increases, we crave protein (carbon, hydrogen, oxygen, and nitrogen); and when we increase our mental activity, we crave carbohydrates (carbon, hydrogen, and oxygen).

The first thing that usually comes to mind when thinking of a nutrient is one or two specific foods from the predominant food group. For example, we think of something sweet for carbohydrates, or meat and eggs for protein. The fact is that most foods contain all six of the major nutrients. The proportion of the nutrients to each other in a specific food is what gives the food a label of either "carbohydrate rich," "protein rich," or "high fat."

The food choices we make each day should be well thought out to keep our bodies healthy and performing efficiently. Eating too much of any one food choice will usually "squeeze out" other food choices. For example, daily consumption of fast foods decreases the chance of consuming more wholesomely prepared foods, and eating sweets throughout the day leaves less appetite for healthier snacks. This is not to say that we should never eat these foods; we just should not eat them exclusively every day or for weeks on end.

The relationship between food and the disease process happens when the body gets too much or too little of a particular nutrient over a period of time. Diabetes, cardiovascular disease, gross obesity, dental caries, and cancer (colon, breast, and reproductive) are major diseases associated with unhealthy eating habits.[6–10] Consistently making unwise food choices can lead to major disease and a shorter lifespan.

🍎 **FOOD FOR THOUGHT 1-1**

The lesson here is that, as humans, we can eat almost anything and still remain healthy, as long as it is in moderation.

PORTION DISTORTION

Researchers discovered that portion sizes in the United States grew in fast food restaurants, the home, and fine dining restaurants over the last 20 years. This increase in portion sizes, coined **portion distortion**, has a direct cause and effect relationship with a rise in obesity. Fast food serving sizes are an average of four times the size they were in the 1950s. Consider the following examples taken from U.S. Department of Health website: http://hp2010.nhlbihin.net/portion/.

Today's fast food cheese burger is 590 calories versus 333 calories 20 years ago. That means one would have to lift weights for 1.5 hours to burn off the additional 257 calories. Hardee's, Burger King, and Wendy's have recently introduced 1,000-plus calorie sandwiches. Twenty years ago, a 2.4 oz serving of french fries had 210 calories. Currently, an average serving of french fries is 6.9 oz for 610 calories—that is 400 more calories! So a meal at a fast food restaurant could add anywhere from 657 to more than 1,000 calories than a similar meal 20 years ago. We should be exercising more than we were 20 years ago to burn off those excess calories, but instead we have become much more sedentary, sitting in front of TVs, computers, and playing video games. We drive instead of walk and let modern appliances do our grunt work. People have a tendency to eat what is in front of them and typically do not calculate the calories. Consumers will equate bigger size with bigger value. **Consumption norm** should be the proper food unit to eat, yet people assume the consumption norm is what is placed before them. If bigger is better when it comes to food presented in a restaurant and at home, then the consumption norm becomes bigger and better. No wonder the average waistline has grown.

No Waste or Small Waist

People have been conditioned from childhood to eat everything on their plate. With the increased size of portions, consumers eat/drink the contents of their meals not until full, but rather until gone. *Either* consumers are not conditioned to be conscious of calories consumed *or* they get more satisfaction from a feeling of getting their money's worth.

Do not be a victim of portion distortion

Opt for the small—forget jumbo, king size, or even large and medium.
Choose water over soda.
Eat half now and the other half later.
Eat slower, savor every bite, and occasionally put the fork down, look around, and see what could happen if you do not become a conscious consumer.

The following is a "snapshot" of American eating culture of 2008. Follow this line of reasoning built from current facts[11]:

Most calories consumed in U.S. diet used to be from white bread. Now it is from soda and sweet drinks. There has been a 14% increase in consumption of sugar and most sweeteners are consumed in soft drinks. Sweets, soft drinks, and alcoholic beverages make up 25% of all calories consumed by Americans while salty snacks and fruit-flavored drinks account for 5% (total of 30%), which means that one-third calories in U.S. diet are junk food. Fifty-one percent of families eat fast food as a family meal one to two times per week and 7% eat fast food dinner meals three to four times per week. Fast food restaurants are the most popular eating establishments for breakfast and lunch and the fast food casual dining is the most popular for dinner. Ease and convenience are top reasons for ordering value/combo meals; yet 50% of consumers would order healthier meals if given a choice, only if they are lower in price.......

🍎 FOOD FOR THOUGHT 1-2

The choice is up to the individual:

No Waste
Portion distortion = over consumption of calories OR
Small Waist
Sensible portion = reasonable consumption of calories

THE FOOD PYRAMID

The U.S. Department of Agriculture (USDA) MyPyramid, shown in Figure 1-1, was designed as a guide to healthy eating and to making healthy food choices. Visit www.mypyramid.gov to set up an individual pyramid food tracker.

Serving suggestions for six food groups have been made to ensure a daily supply of important nutrients. It should be remembered that MyPyramid guidelines are suggestions and can be modified to accommodate specific diet requirements, such as those for people who are vegetarians, who are lactose intolerant, or who have specific cultural and religious practices. According to MyPyramid, we should include various foods from each category, considering the following while doing so:

- Three rich sources of calcium
- Three high protein foods

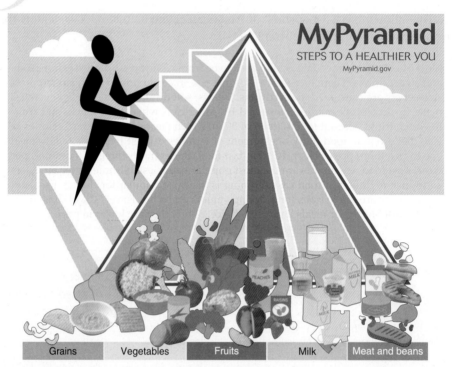

| Grains | Vegetables | Fruits | Milk | Meat and beans |

FIGURE 1-1   MyPyramid: a guide to daily food choices. (Reprinted from the U.S. Department of Agriculture and the U.S. Department of Health and Human Services. 6th ed. 2007. See Mypyramid.gov.)

- At least five servings of vegetables and fruits
- Whole grains for fiber
- Vegetable fats and omega-3 fatty acids

Add to that at least eight glasses of water and moderate exercise, and you have a plan to maintain a healthy body. (See Chapter 11 for more detail on the MyPyramid.)

FOOD HABITS

We may be choosing the food we eat out of habit or because we have a physiologic need for certain nutrients. Some **food habits** have specific origins. They can be born out of family traditions—like turkey for Thanksgiving, cake on birthdays, and cookies for Christmas. Other habits are created because of the way food makes us feel, especially when we are stressed or upset. Foods high in fat and carbohydrates tend to be chosen as comfort foods.[12,13] A physiologic need for certain foods—also considered a craving—can turn into a true habit if not met. Social occasions add to our habits with their cyclic list of foods to serve, for example, veggies and dip, sushi, and other finger foods.

Reasons for Food Habits

It has been said that the human body has an innate wisdom and will let us know when it requires a specific nutrient or chemical, and that when we have a craving *whether or not true* our body is talking to us. Whether or not this is true, the fact is that **food cravings** can be either emotional or physiologic. Not everybody gets them, but for those who do, they are very real. If our craving is on an emotional level, then the craving remains as long as the emotional need remains. If we fulfill the need, then the craving goes away.

A physiologic hormone fluctuation can trigger a food craving, which is why they are reported more by women than men. Cravings can turn into a full-blown habit that needs to be fed on a daily basis. Sometimes they are a steady constant, like having ice cream every night after dinner. We can go through phases, like eating peanut butter and crackers every day around 4:00 PM for 2 weeks, and then smoked almonds at the same time for the next 2 weeks. This is neither accidental nor coincidental. If what we crave is based on a physiologic need, then our bodies will let us know when they are balanced and no longer need the chemical.

What are our bodies trying to tell us when we have a craving? Usually one of the following four things:

1. We need a mood adjustment—levels of neurotransmitters are fluctuating and we require the need to obtain balance with a nutrient from the specific food we crave.
2. Our blood sugar level is low and carbohydrates are needed to boost energy level. *blood sugar*
3. We are lacking a specific nutrient and the food we crave will balance body chemistry.
4. Something is out of balance emotionally and comfort food is desired to help us cope.

Here are some ideas to minimize a food craving:

- Move your body—exercise, stretch, or practice yoga to stave off depressive feelings.
- Choose complex carbohydrates for meals that will moderate blood sugar levels throughout the day.

- Eat frequent small nutritious meals throughout the day. This will minimize the sensation of being hungry.
- Give in and eat a modest amount of what is craved.

🍎 FOOD FOR THOUGHT 1-3

Chocolate is the single-most craved food.[14] Some say it is not even food, but rather medicine because it contains phenylethylamine, a mood enhancer, and caffeinelike substances called "methylxanthine" and "theobromine." Eating chocolate balances brain chemicals and boosts energy.

Take a moment and think about your reasons for eating the foods you do. Pay attention to your body to determine if specific foods can change how you feel. When you feel like eating a snack, such as potato chips or candy, ask yourself if you are truly hungry, or if you are bored, upset, anxious, or tired. Identifying

TABLE 1-1   Influence of Food

Keep a record of how your food selections make you feel. Check in with your body 30 minutes after consuming a particular food to determine what it does.

Food	Energetic	Happy	Clear mind	Disoriented	Sleepy	Depressed
bagle cream cheese		✓			✓	
tomatoes	✓	✓				
banana					✓	

the feeling before you eat can help you understand your eating habits. Make an inventory list of your favorite food selections and see if you can identify your comfort foods. Then complete Table 1-1 and see if foods you choose affect you in a certain way.

DIGESTIVE PROCESS

The **gastrointestinal (GI) tract**, which supplies the body with nutrients and water, includes the following hollow organs:

1. Esophagus
2. Stomach
3. Small intestine
4. Large intestine
5. Rectum

Three other solid organs—pancreas, liver, and gallbladder (along with the small intestine)—secrete enzymes that help reduce the food to micronutrients (Figure 1-2).

The digestive process begins even before food or drink reaches the mouth. Low blood sugar level and our sense of smell can stimulate our desire for food and drink. Just thinking about eating can wake up resting digestive organs and get the "juices flowing." The food and drink we put into our mouths is not in a form that the body can use as nourishment, so it must go through a very complex process before nutrients can do their thing, such as provide energy, repair injured tissue, boost immune system, and make body cells and tissue. Digestion is an integrated process that requires team work from our body's voluntary and involuntary nervous systems that begins in the mouth, continues in the small intestines where most absorption of nutrients takes place, and ends in the large intestine where solid waste is excreted. We voluntarily put the food and drink in our mouths, rip and grind with our teeth, and swallow the soft mashed up food, but once it leaves the oral cavity, it is up to involuntary forces to guide the food through the rest of its journey.

The act of chewing reduces food to smaller particles, making it easier to swallow and pass through to the stomach. The human dentition crushes food with a force of almost 200 lb (90 kg), mashing the bolus of food, mixing it with enzymes excreted from salivary glands. The ability to chew well is vital to the digestive process because this is the first step in preparing food for enzyme action. Aside from breaking up food into smaller parts, the act of chewing causes

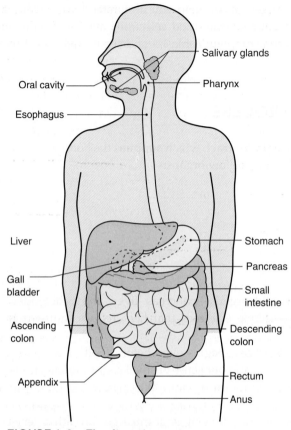

FIGURE 1-2   **The digestive system.**

involuntary secretion of enzymes from the pancreas, liver, gall bladder, and small intestine. Patients with limited chewing ability may complain of digestive problems, which is why they need to be encouraged to replace missing teeth and correct temporomandibular joint (TMJ) disorders.

Enzymes are of vital importance during the digestive process because they rearrange and divide food molecules, making them more bioavailable to the human body. If it were not for enzymes, nutrients in food could not be used by the body. Digestive enzymes are specifically designed to do one particular job. Major enzyme groups are named to represent the job they do or the food they work on: protease works on protein, lipase works on lipids, and amylase works on carbohydrates. An amylase called "ptyalin" is the first to be secreted in the digestive process, produced by salivary glands to break apart starch molecules into maltose. Sucrase breaks down sucrose and lactase breaks down lactose. If a body lacks an enzyme, then that individual will be intolerant to the food it works on; lack of lactase would make someone unable to drink milk because of milk sugar called "lactose." (See Chapter 2 and section "Lactose Intolerance.") Sometimes it may take more than one type of enzyme to break apart food, as is the case with process of breaking apart protein. A protease called "pepsin," secreted by the stomach, breaks protein into polypeptides, then the process is continued by another protease called "trypsin," manufactured by the pancreas, which continues to break down the protein while it is in the small intestine.

As the body ages its ability to produce enzymes diminishes, which limits nutrient absorption. Elderly patients may report the use of food enzymes which helps with the digestion of all types of food. Emotional and mental strain can also influence production of enzymes, lending more credence to suggestions for positive, calm eating experience.

After food has been chewed, swallowing pushes the food into the esophagus, the "hallway" that funnels food into the stomach by way of **peristalsis** (alternating contractions and relaxation), until it hits the sphincter, the "door" that will open and admit the food to the stomach. The stomach stores the masticated food for about 1.5 hours and continues to break it down into smaller particles with the aid of the enzyme pepsin and hydrochloric acid, which is secreted by the gastric gland. The contents being held in the stomach—food bolus, enzymes, and acids—have been turned into a mixture called "chyme," which continues the journey into the small intestines. At this point, the liver produces bile to assist with breaking down fat and protein. The action of bile on fat and protein is similar to that of a degreaser. Proteins, carbohydrates, fats, vitamins, minerals, water, and alcohol have all been reduced to the smallest unit possible so that they can permeate the intestinal wall and find their way into the bloodstream.

🍎 FOOD FOR THOUGHT 1-4

Why does hydrochloric acid not destroy the lining of the stomach? Hydrochloric acid is an aqueous solution of hydrogen chloride and gastric acid that protects us from harmful bacteria we may ingest with our food and harmful bacteria that may migrate from the colon into small intestines. The stomach and intestines are lined with a healthy amount of bicarbonate-containing mucus, which protects organ linings from the effects of this caustic acid. Its industrial name is "muriatic acid." It can burn a hole if poured on wood. Some uses are to etch concrete, clean lime residue, and process leather.

The small intestine is divided into three sections: duodenum, jejunum, and ileum. Most digestion and absorption takes place in the small intestines, more specifically the jejunum. The lining of the intestines is variegated rather than smooth, with peaks called "villi." The villi extensions increase the surface area of the small intestines, allowing for quicker passage of nutrients (3 to 10 hours). Once these small units of digested food pass into the bloodstream, they travel to all parts of the body, supplying it with fuel and nutrients needed for all metabolic processes.

Remnants of food that did not digest become waste and pass on to the large intestine, where water is absorbed from the waste, turning it to solid feces. Unlike the small intestine, the lining of the large intestine is smooth. Bacteria in the feces can manufacture vitamin K and biotin, which can be absorbed and used by the body.

The rectum stores the feces until our brain gets the signal to eliminate it. Total "intestinal transit time" can be anywhere from 24 hours to 3 weeks.

🍎 FOOD FOR THOUGHT 1-5

Hormones that regulate appetite:
Ghrelin is an appetite stimulant that is produced in the stomach and upper intestine in the absence of food.

Peptide YY is an appetite suppression hormone produced in the small intestine and colon in response to eating a full meal.

CURRENT AND FUTURE NUTRITION TRENDS

According to the American Dietetic Association, there are two kinds of nutrition trends; those that develop from a slow-growing groundswell as from a new book or scientific research that then saturates the market, and those that occur from a milestone, like people dying from a foodborne disease. Most nutrition trends are from the first category with people jumping on the bandwagon as TV and magazines inundate the population with information. One year, the no-carbohydrate Atkins diet was the best diet advice, and the next year people were strongly reminded about the benefits of complex carbohydrates. Just as all other trends come and go, so do many widely publicized nutritional trends. Currently gaining popularity are:

1. Functional foods—food that is fortified with abundant nutrients like vitamins, minerals, lutein, flavonoids, and isoflavones. Examples would

be the addition of calcium to orange juice and flavonoids in grape juice and red wine.

2. Eating "green" by choosing locally grown organic foods that are kinder to the environment by using less fossil fuel to grow, process, and bring to market. Certified organically grown food also limits exposures to harmful pesticides, herbicides, and other chemicals used in traditional farming practices. Buying locally also gives the product a nutritional edge by being picked when ripe and nutrient dense. Produce picked at factory farms is harvested before ripe and then travels 4 to 7 days before displaying in grocery stores, reducing up to 50% of its nutrients.

3. Single-serve packaging that limits the amount of calories consumed in one sitting, making the consumption norm a lower calorie choice.

4. Bottled vitamin water to boost the nutrients consumed in the daily diet.

Current social events will also prompt new areas of study. Since the 9/11 event, scientists are searching for ways to assure protection of our food crops from terrorist attacks. And with all the concern of global warming, there is an urgent need to develop ways to produce more food using less water and studying climate gas disruption of the food chain.

Scientific research continues to turn up new ideas that provoke curious thought leading to new studies. As our world evolves and population preferences shift, technology develops to serve the needs of the scientific community. As in all other disciplines, the study of nutrition will always have its share of careful observers who remain on the cutting edge, willing to bring the most current information to the masses.

Putting This Into Practice

The goal of this project is to jump-start your mind to begin thinking about nutrition and its relation to the body.

Your assignment is to visit a grocery store of your choice with a relative or friend and passively observe their food choices and food selection process.

Answer the following questions about your observations:

1. List the food items in your selected person's shopping cart.

(continued)

2. What body type do they have? Circle one:

    Ectomorphic—light body build with slight muscular development
    Mesomorphic—husky muscular body build
    Endomorphic—heavy rounded body build often with a marked
       tendency to become fat

3. Does their body type match the food they have chosen
   to eat? Explain.
4. Who or what do you think they were shopping for?
5. What would you add to their selection to balance out their diet?
6. What would you eliminate from their selection to make their diet more
   nutritious?
7. Did they read labels as they chose food for their carts?
8. Draw a conclusion about food choices and our bodies.

WEB RESOURCES

American Dietetic Association (ADA) www.eatright.org

The Blonz Guide to Nutrition, Food Science, and Health www.blonz.com

CDC's Nutrition and Physical Activity www.cdc.gov/nccdphp/dnpa

ENC: Egg Nutrition Center www.enc-online.org

Food and Nutrition Information Center www.nal.usda.gov/fnic

Government Information on Nutrition www.nutrition.gov

Harvard School of Public Health www.hsph.harvard.edu

Journal of Nutrition www.nutrition.org

Nutrition Action Health Letter www.cspinet.org/nah/index.htm

Nutrition and Healthy Eating Advice www.nutrition.about.com

Tufts University Nutrition Navigator: A Rating Guide to Nutrition Websites
    www.navigator.tufts.edu

Untangling the Web– How to Find Useful Nutrition and Health Information On Line
    http://cspinet.org/nah/2003/untangling_the_web.html

The Vegetarian Resource Group www.vrg.org/nutrition

Eating at Fast Food Restaurants More Than Twice Per Week is Associated With More
    Weight Gain and Insulin Resistance in Otherwise Healthy Adults
    http://www.nih.gov/news/pr/dec2004/nhlbi_30.htm

Portion Distortion http://hin.nhlbi.nih.gov/portion

http://hp2010.nhlbihin.net/portion/

Guide to Healthy Fast Food Restaurant Eating www.helpguide.org/life/fast_food_nutrition.htm

UNC Study Confirms That Food Portion Sizes Increased in US Over Two Decades
www.sciencedaily.com/releases/2003/01/030122072329.htm

(JAMA Jan 2nd) science daily 22 January 2003.5 January 2008

REFERENCES

1. Schlosser E. *Fast Food Nation: The Dark Side of the All American Meal*. Boston: Houghton Mifflin; 2000.
2. Popkin BM. Nutrition in transition: the changing global nutrition challenge. *Asia Pac. J. Clin. Nutr*. 2001;10(Suppl):S13–S18.
3. Blake J. *Measuring Our Dining, Shopping Habits—Survey Finds We Like to Eat Out, Shop Around (Survey from Market Research Firm NPD Foodworld)*: Seattle Times; Feb. 11, 2003.
4. Ebbin R. *American's dining out habits*. Restaurants USA, November 2000.
5. Tougher-Decker R, Mobley CC. American Dietetic Association. Position of the American Dietetic Association: oral health and nutrition. *J. Am. Diet. Assoc*. 2003;103(5): 615–625.
6. Key TJ, Schatzkin A, Willett WC, et al. Diet, nutrition and the prevention of cancer. *Public Health Nutr*. 2004;7(1A):187–200.
7. Vandewater EA, Shim MS, Caplovitz AG. Linking obesity and activity level with children's television and video game use. *J. Adolesc*. 2004;27(1):71–85.
8. Simonpoulos AP. The traditional diet of Greece and cancer. *Eur. J. Cancer Prev*. 2004; 13:219–230.
9. Cannon G. Why the Bush administration and the global sugar industry are determined to demolish the 2004 WHO global strategy on diet, physical activity and health. *Public Health Nutr*. 2004;7(3):369–380.
10. Proietto J, Baur LA. 10: management of obesity. *Med. J. Aust*. 2004;180(9):474–480.
11. Mayer J. USDA Human Nutrition Research Center on aging at Tufts University and Gladys Brock. *J Public Health Nutr*. 2007.
12. Pelchat ML. Of human bondage: food craving, obsession, compulsion, and addiction. *Physiol. Behav*. 2002;76(3):347–352.
13. Yanovski S. Sugar and fat: cravings and aversions. *J. Nutr*. 2003;133(3):835 S–837 S.
14. Rice S, McAllister EJ, Dhurandhar NV. Fast food friendly? *Int. J. Obes*. 2007;31(6): 884–886.

SUGGESTED READING

Christensen L, Pettijohn L. Mood and carbohydrate cravings. *Appetite* 2001;36(2):137–145.

Cohen D, Farley TA. Eating as an automatic behavior. *Prev. Chronic Dis*. 2008;5(1):A23.

Hill AJ, Weaver CF, Blundell JE. Food craving, dietary restraint and mood. *Appetite* 1991; 17(3):187–197.

Matthiessen J, Fagt S, Biltoft-Jensen A, et al. Size makes a difference. *Public Health Nutr.* 2003;6(1):65–72.

Raynor HA, Wing RR. Package unit size and amount of food: do both influence intake? *Obesity (Silver Spring)* 2007;15(9):2311–2319.

Rodd HD, Patel V. Content analysis of children's television advertising in relation to dental health. *Braz. Dent. J.* 2005;199(11):710–712.

Smiciklas-Wright H, Mitchell DC, Mickle SJ, et al. Foods commonly eaten in the United States, 1989–1991 and 1994–1996: are portion sizes changing? *J. Am. Diet. Assoc.* 2003; 103(1):39–40.

Wansink B, Cheney MM, Chan N. Exploring comfort food preferences across age and gender. *Physiol. Behav.* 2003;79(4-5):739–747.

Weingarten HP, Elston D. The phenomenology of food cravings. *Appetite* 1990;15(3): 231–246.

Wilson N, Quigley R, Mansoor O. Food ads on TV: a health hazard for children? *Aust. N Z J. Public Health* 1999;23(6):647–650.

Zellner DA, Garriga-Trillo A, Rohm E, et al. Food liking and craving: a cross-cultural approach. *Appetite* 1999;33(1):61–70.

MAJOR NUTRIENTS

Major Nutrients AT A GLANCE

Major Nutrient	Molecular Structure	Primary Role in Body	Source in Diet	Recommended Dietary Intake	Digestion/Absorption	Kcal/g[a]
Carbohydrate	$C_6H_{12}O_6$	Energy Maintain steady blood glucose levels Spare Proteins Provide bulk	Grains Fruits Vegetables Dairy	45%–55% of total daily calories	Begins in mouth when mixed with amylase and continues with pancreatic amylase in small intestines; passes through wall of small intestines where absorbed by body	4
Protein	COOH (carboxyl group) NH_2 (amino radical) Carbon and hydrogen side group	Growth Maintenance Repair	Meat Diary	40–65 g/day depending on weight	Begins in stomach when mixed with pepsin, passes to small intestines where it mixes with trypsin and chymotrypsin; passes through wall of small intestines where absorbed by body	4
Lipid	Carbon atom with carboxyl end (COOH) And methyl end (CH_3)	Insulate against cold Cushions orgains Energy Cell structure Provides fat soluble vitamins	Meat Dairy Butter and oil Sauces and salad dressing	<30% total daily calories	Begins in mouth when mixed with lipase and continues in stomach when mixed with gastric lipase; emulsified by bile and pancreatic lipase in small intestines; passes through wall of small intestines where absorbed by body	9

Continued on next page

Major Nutrients AT A GLANCE (continued)

Major Nutrient	Molecular Structure	Primary Role in Body	Source in Diet	Recommended Dietary Intake	Digestion/Absorption	Kcal/g[a]
Vitamins	Varied	Releases energy from food	Fortified foods / Fruits and vegetables / Animal foods	Varies	Released from food but not digested; cycles through digestive process with food; permeates wall of small intestines; water soluble vitamins that are not used are excreted, fat soluble not used are stored in fat depots	0
Minerals	Varied	Controls water balance / Nerve transmission / Muscle contractions / Tissue synthesis / Energy balance / Facilitates antioxidan process	Unrefined foods / Food grown in rich soil and from oceans	Varies	Released from food but not digested; cycles through digestive process with food; permeates wall of small intestine and are absorbed by the body or transported out in waste	0
Water	H_2O	Solvent for metabolic processes / Removes toxins / Transports nutrients / Builds tissue / Regulates temperature / Cushions organs / Lubricates mucous membranes	Drinking water / Liquid Beverages / Food	64 oz	Freely passes through small intestine membranes and is absorbed; can be reabsorbed by the colon	0

[a]See Chapter 12.

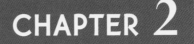

CHAPTER 2

CARBOHYDRATES

OBJECTIVES

Upon completion of this chapter, the reader will be able to:

1 Name the categories of chemical and nutritive classifications of carbohydrates

2 Discuss the difference between monosaccharide, disaccharide, and polysaccharide

3 Explain the digestive process of carbohydrates in the body

4 Describe maintenance of blood glucose level and outline the steps involved in reducing excess glucose and making glucose available when the level is low

5 Differentiate between an insoluble and soluble fiber

6 Explain what happens in the body when carbohydrates are restricted from the diet

7 Give examples of foods that are rich in fiber and discuss their importance in the diet

8 Counsel patients about the benefits of carbohydrates in the diet and guide them to choose those that are complex versus simple

KEY TERMS

Complex Carbohydrate
Disaccharide
Glycemic Index
Insoluble

Ketosis
Monosaccharide
Oligosaccharide
Polysaccharide

Roughage
Satiety
Simple Sugar
Soluble

Carbohydrates AT A GLANCE

Molecular Structure	Primary Role in Body	Source in Diet	Recommended Dietary Intake	Digestion/Absorption	Kcal/gm
$C_6H_{12}O_6$	Energy Maintain steady blood glucose levels Spare protein Provide bulk	Grains, fruits, vegetables, and dairy products	45%–55% total daily calories	Begins in mouth when mixed with amylase, passes through wall of small intestines and absorbed by body	4

Before the Industrial Revolution, carbohydrates (CHO) were the greatest proportion of foods consumed and therefore the main source of nutrients. Geographically, regions had their own staple food that was indigenous to their land. These staple foods (carbohydrates) were consumed in the whole or natural form (without processing) and considered rich with vitamins, minerals, and fiber. Table 2-1 identifies the food staple by region.

Along with the Industrial Revolution came the invention of a machine for everything, including one for processing wheat, sugarcane, and sugar beets into a refined white powder. To get the fine white powder, the husks and pulp had to be removed, which was the part of the plant that contained all the nutrients and fiber. Because these were removed, the powdered flour and sugar lost nutritive value but retained calories. It was considered a luxury and a display of wealth to

TABLE 2-1	Main Food Staples by Region
Asia	Rice
Middle East	Wheat
Great Britain	Barley and oats
Pacific Islands	Taro root
Africa	Cassava root and yams
America	Potatoes and corn

have a pantry full of bleached white flour and sugar, and its owner usually had a growing belly to prove it. What once were wealthy sources of nutrients became poor sources, but the consumption of them remained the same. People began to load their meals with "refined" ingredients, which corresponded to an increase in incidence of obesity. This is how carbohydrates got a bad reputation of being fattening. Many years ago the connection was proven false as it was discovered that all the "extras" eaten with the meal, not the carbohydrates, are what caused the increase in obesity. Butter, sour cream, salad dressing, and added sugars such as jellies, jams, and syrup are now recognized as the fat-producing culprits. Carbohydrates, when carefully selected, can actually be an excellent low-fat source of fiber and nutrients.

When asked, most people will reply that carbohydrates are sugar. In essence, they are half right. Carbohydrates are a *type* of sugar, but all carbohydrates are not sweet like table sugar. Rice, pasta, bread, fruits, and vegetables are also considered carbohydrates. The size of the chemical arrangement is what determines the flavor, but they all do pretty much the same thing in the body.

CARBOHYDRATES IN THE ECOSYSTEM

With the exception of one sugar, plants are the source of all carbohydrates. Figure 2-1 illustrates where CHOs fit into the food chain.

Food Chain

1. Plant roots absorb water.
2. Foliage absorbs carbon dioxide (CO_2) from the air.
3. Plant absorbs rays from the sun.
4. Chloroplasts in the plant take all three—H_2O, sun, and CO_2—and through photosynthesis make monosaccharides.
5. Animals eat the plant and reduce the monosaccharides to glucose.

PRIMARY ROLE OF CARBOHYDRATES IN THE BODY

The primary roles of carbohydrates are to:

- Supply the body with energy
- Maintain blood glucose levels

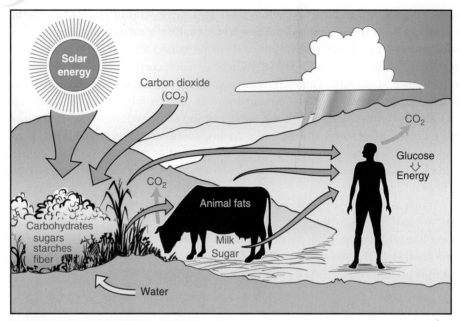

FIGURE 2-1   The carbon cycle.

- Continue brain and nervous system function, even while sleeping
- Spare protein so the body does not burn dietary or body fat and protein for energy
- Burn fat for fuel
- Provide bulk in the diet (fiber) and keep you full

Food for Thought 2-1 identifies the only CHO of animal origin.

🍎 **FOOD FOR THOUGHT 2-1**

Lactose (milk sugar) is the only carbohydrate of animal origin.

CLASSIFICATION OF CARBOHYDRATES

The word "carbohydrate" is Latin for hydrated water. Carbohydrates are often abbreviated to CHO for the three elements that comprise it: carbon, hydrogen,

TABLE 2-2 Classification of Carbohydrates	
Chemical	Nutritional
Monosaccharide	Simple carbohydrate
Disaccharide	—
Oligosaccharide	Complex carbohydrate
Polysaccharide	—

and oxygen. The chemical building blocks of CHOs are called "monosaccharides," which are composed of 6 carbon, 12 hydrogen, and 6 oxygen atoms ($C_6H_{12}O_6$). Generally speaking, there are two ways to classify CHOs: Table 2-2 outlines these two classification systems.

The chemical classification helps us understand how the molecules of carbohydrates link together, and the nutritional classification determines their value in our diet.

Chemical Classification of Carbohydrates

The main unit of carbohydrate is a monosaccharide (glucose molecule). One molecule of glucose consists of 6 carbon atoms, 12 hydrogen atoms, and 6 oxygen atoms: $C_6H_{12}O_6$. Figures 2-2 and 2-3 illustrate the chemical structures of monosaccharides and disaccharides, respectively.

1. **Monosaccharide**: one molecule of sugar
2. **Disaccharide**: two molecules of sugar
3. **Oligosaccharide**: 2 to 10 molecules of sugar
4. **Polysaccharide**: more than 10 molecules of sugar

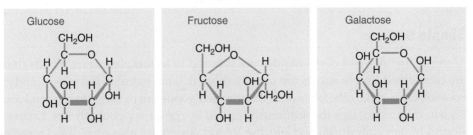

FIGURE 2-2   Chemical structure of monosaccharides.

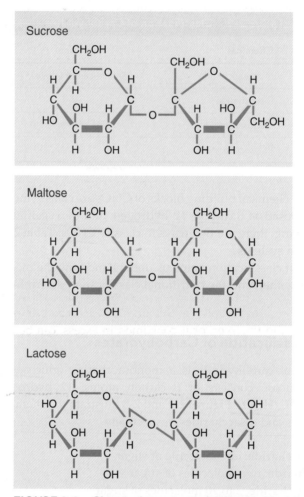

FIGURE 2-3   Chemical structure of disaccharides.

NUTRITIONAL CLASSIFICATION OF CARBOHYDRATES

Simple Sugars

Monosaccharides and disaccharides are referred to as **simple sugars**. Foods that are considered simple sugars are usually those that are sweet to the taste. Candy, cookies, cake, soda, ripe fruits, and other baked goods fall in this category and are high in calories but lack the nutrients supplied by complex carbohydrates. Lactose (found in dairy products) and glucose (blood sugar) are also considered simple sugars, but are not sweet to the taste.

TABLE 2-3 Simple Carbohydrates and Complex Carbohydrates	
Simple Carbohydrate	**Complex Carbohydrate**
White bread	Whole grain bread
White rice	Brown rice
Semolina pasta	Whole wheat pasta
Sugar-sweetened juices	100% fruit juice and vegetable juice
Flour tortillas	Wheat or spinach tortillas

Table 2-3 lists common monosaccharides, disaccharides, and polysaccharides.

Monosaccharides

1. Glucose (also called "dextrose" or "blood sugar") is the main currency for the body's fuel source that supplies energy. Most other sugars are either converted or broken down to this unit. Glucose can be stored as glycogen in muscle and the liver, or if consumed in excess, can be converted to fat for future energy supply.
2. Fructose is the sweetest of all sugars and found in fruit and honey. It is converted by the body to glucose.
3. Galactose, also known as "milk sugar," is converted by the body to glucose.

Disaccharides

1. Sucrose (also known as "table sugar") consists of the monosaccharides glucose and fructose, which make table sugar sweet. This is used in cooking and baking for a sweet taste.
2. Maltose consists of two glucose molecules and is created when larger carbohydrate molecules are broken down during digestion.
3. Lactose, the sugar found in milk, splits into the two monosaccharides glucose and galactose during digestion.

Complex Carbohydrates

Polysaccharides are referred to as **complex carbohydrates**. Foods high in complex carbohydrates contain vitamins, minerals, fiber, and water. Brown rice, whole grain bread, cereal, whole wheat pasta, legumes, fruits, and vegetables are foods rich in complex carbohydrates. Complex carbohydrates supply more nutrients than simple carbohydrates and are a very good low-fat food source. Food for Thought 2-2 lists common polysaccharides.

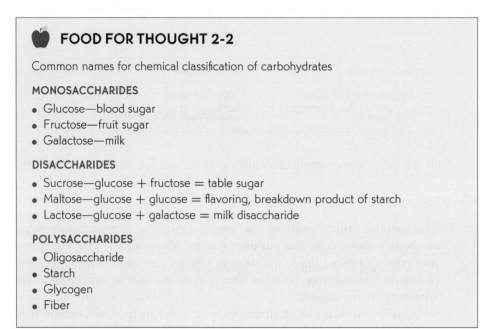

🍎 FOOD FOR THOUGHT 2-2

Common names for chemical classification of carbohydrates

MONOSACCHARIDES

- Glucose—blood sugar
- Fructose—fruit sugar
- Galactose—milk

DISACCHARIDES

- Sucrose—glucose + fructose = table sugar
- Maltose—glucose + glucose = flavoring, breakdown product of starch
- Lactose—glucose + galactose = milk disaccharide

POLYSACCHARIDES

- Oligosaccharide
- Starch
- Glycogen
- Fiber

Oligosaccharides

Oligosaccharides are a unique type of carbohydrate because the body does not metabolize them in the usual way. They are larger than a disaccharide—at least two or more single sugar molecules—and are found in legumes (beans). Oligosaccharides pass through the stomach undigested into the intestines, where bacteria feed on the carbohydrate and create a gaseous end product (which gives beans their bad reputation).

Starch

Starch is the storage form of energy in plants, just as glycogen is the storage form of energy in animals. The arrangement of glucose molecules determines whether the starch is amylose or amylopectin, the two most predominant starches.

Amylopectin is a series of highly branched chains of glucose molecules. It is sometimes referred to as a "waxy starch" that forms a stringy paste when heated, and this property makes it work well as a thickener in food. Amylose is composed of thousands of straight-chain glucose molecules. Foods that contain starch are grains, legumes, tubers (potatoes, yams, and turnips), and some fruits.

See which foods you eat contain starch by performing the simple experiment detailed in Food for Thought 2-3.

🍎 FOOD FOR THOUGHT 2-3

EXPERIMENT WITH YOUR FOOD

One way to tell if a food contains starch is to add a drop of iodine. The unbranched helical shape of amylose reacts strongly to iodine and turns it blue-black. Amylopectin, cellulose, and glycogen will turn the iodine reddish-purple and brown.

Starch is used as a thickening agent in cooking and baking. A good example is cornstarch: When mixed with water over heat, it forms a sauce or gravy. When we consume starch, it gives us a sense of **satiety** or fullness, and the sense of being full stays with us for a longer period of time.

Food for Thought 2-4 outlines the digestion of starch.

🍎 FOOD FOR THOUGHT 2-4

DIGESTION OF STARCH

- Salivary amylase in the mouth breaks starch down to dextrins.
- Pancreatic amylase in the small intestine breaks dextrins down to maltose.
- Maltase splits maltose into glucose units, which can be absorbed.

Glucose

Glycogen is the most highly branched chain of glucose units and is the storage form of carbohydrates that is found in the liver and muscle.

In liver—helps maintain blood glucose levels
In muscle—provides quick supply of energy for muscles

Fiber

Fiber is the food that is usually referred to as **roughage** or "bulk" and is not used by the body for energy. Fiber is thousands of glucose units bonded together and is found exclusively in plants, giving them structure. Fiber in plants is equal to bones in animals. A good example of fiber is the stringy strips that run the length of celery.

See Food for Thought 2-5

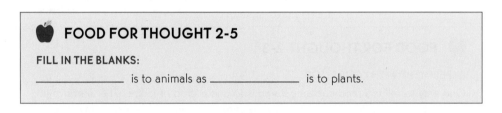

🍎 FOOD FOR THOUGHT 2-5

FILL IN THE BLANKS:

_____ is to animals as _____ is to plants.

Humans do not have enzymes that can break down and digest fiber. The chemical links between fiber molecules are joined in such a way that they cannot be separated by human digestive enzymes. Vitamins and minerals in fiber-rich foods are not made available to the body and pass through unabsorbed. See Figure 2-4 for an illustration of enzyme activity. There are two general classes of fiber.

Soluble Fiber—Dissolves in Water

- Examples are gums, mucilage, and pectin, as in the gelatinous substance that forms in cooked oatmeal.
- Foods high in soluble fiber are fruits, vegetables, grains, beans, oats, and apples.

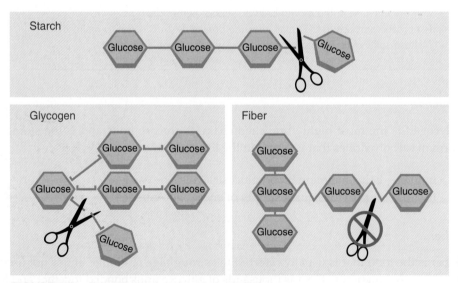

FIGURE 2-4   Enzymes cannot break apart fiber.

Function of Soluble Fiber
- Adds chewy or crunchy texture to foods
- Gives a sense of satiety—keeps the stomach full longer
- Stabilizes blood sugar—takes longer for the body to metabolize and slows release of glucose into bloodstream
- Helps lower cholesterol—binds fiber and carries it out of the body in waste

Insoluble Fiber—does not Dissolve in Water

- Insoluble fiber is found in seeds.
- Other examples are cellulose and lignin, such as the stringy strips in celery. Cellulose is the most abundant polysaccharide.
- Foods high in insoluble fiber are vegetables, whole grains, wheat bran, and apples.

Function of Insoluble Fiber
Insoluble fiber prevents disease by stimulating peristalsis and keeps colon muscles exercised and strong. Fiber also acts to decrease:
- Constipation
- Hemorrhoids
- Diverticulosis (outpouchings in colon wall)/diverticulitis (infected out-pouchings)
- Colon cancer—empties the colon so that lining of intestines and colon are not exposed to toxins for a long period of time
- Incidence of appendicitis

TABLE 2-4	Grams of Fiber in Food		
Food	Total Fiber	Soluble Fiber	Insoluble Fiber
Oat bran	28	14	14
Rolled oats	14	8	6
Wheat bran	43	3	40
Kidney beans	10	5	5
Pinto beans	11	5	6
Corn	3	2	1
Apple	2	1	1
Orange	2	1	1

Table 2-4 lists the grams of the different types of fiber found in certain foods. When increasing the amount of fiber in your diet, do so gradually to allow your body time to adapt. Increasing the amount too fast will result in waste elimination problems. Drink plenty of fluids to keep stools hydrated, allowing for less constipation.

MAINTENANCE OF BLOOD GLUCOSE HOMEOSTASIS

Normal blood glucose is 80 to 100 mg/dL of blood. When blood glucose is higher, you have *hyperglycemia* (*over*). When blood glucose is lower, you have *hypoglycemia* (*under*).

Insulin and glucagon are the two hormones involved in maintaining blood glucose levels. When the body has too much blood glucose, we feel an excess of energy and are nervous and excitable. When there is not enough blood glucose, we can feel lethargic, disoriented, and confused. Maintaining the right amount of glucose in the blood is called "homeostasis." When the amount of glucose in our blood is in balance with what our body needs, we have an overall sense of well-being and feel just the right amount of energy and alertness. Table sugar and foods rich in simple sugars will overdose our system with glucose, giving us the feeling of both extremes in a short period of time. This is called "spiking" (loading our bodies with sugar) and is a harmful pattern. We feel a rapid surge of energy and a rapid decline in energy in a short time span. When we feel the drop in energy, the first inclination is to eat a candy bar or drink a soda to feel energetic again. This behavior greatly increases the amount of calories ingested (with no nutrients) and lends itself to detrimental long-term effects such as obesity and dental caries. Homeostasis works as follows (and is illustrated in Figure 2-5):

1. Receptor cells in the pancreas recognize that there is more glucose in the blood than the body currently needs for energy. The pancreas secretes the hormone insulin, which draws out the excess glucose, thus reducing the amount of blood glucose when the level gets too high. It attracts glucose from the bloodstream and stores it in the muscle and the liver, where it is converted to glycogen. The glycogen stays in the muscle until the body needs it for energy to move the muscle, and then it is stored in the liver for future energy use. There is a limit to the capacity of glycogen storing cells:
   • Once the stores are filled, the overflow is routed to fat.
   • Fat cells enlarge and fill with fat.
   • Fat cell storage capacity is unlimited.

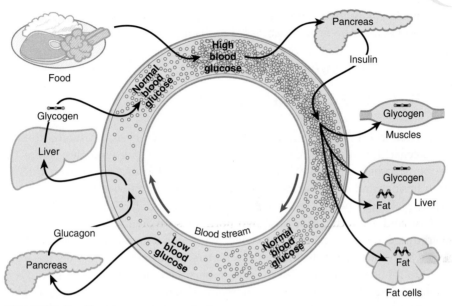

FIGURE 2-5   Blood sugar homeostasis.

2. Receptor cells in the pancreas recognize that the body is in need of energy so the pancreas secretes the hormone glucagon, which converts the glycogen in the liver to glucose and releases it into the bloodstream, where it is carried through the body and used for fuel.

How the Body Regulates Blood Sugar

- Eating carbohydrates throughout the day will help maintain blood glucose levels. Eat a little with each meal.
- Whenever possible, choose the whole grain version of the food, because it is metabolized more slowly by the body.
- Avoid refined sugars—they are empty calories.

RECOMMENDED DIETARY INTAKE

There is no recommended dietary intake for carbohydrates, but it has been loosely recommended at 55% to 65% of total daily calorie intake, with 25 g to 35 g being fiber. This amounts to about 300 g for a sedentary person and 500 g for a physically active person. It has also been suggested that we limit daily intake of refined sugar to less than 20% of total calorie intake, which includes the sugar present in processed foods like jams, jellies, baked goods, and beverages.

DIGESTION OF CARBOHYDRATES

Monosaccharides do not require breakdown by enzymes, but disaccharides and polysaccharides must be reduced to monosaccharides by enzymes before they can be absorbed and used by the body. Polysaccharides are broken down to disaccharides and disaccharides are broken down to monosaccharides. The splitting of molecules begins in the mouth when polysaccharides mix with salivary amylase and are reduced to disaccharides. Further degradation happens when the reduced molecules come in contact with stomach acids. Disaccharides are passed into the small intestine, where pancreatic amylase completes the breakdown to monosaccharides. These small monosaccharides then pass through the small intestinal villi into the bloodstream, where they travel to the liver for nutrient processing before being sent out to all parts of the body for use as energy.

Food for Thought 2-6 indicates enzyme breakdown of disaccharides to monosaccharides.

🍎 FOOD FOR THOUGHT 2-6

- Sucrose is broken down by sucrase into glucose and fructose.
- Maltose is broken down by maltase into glucose units.
- Lactose is broken down by lactase into glucose and galactose.

GLYCEMIC INDEX

Glycemic Index is a numeric ranking system for carbohydrates based on their immediate effect on blood glucose levels. Foods high in fats and protein do not cause the rise in blood sugar levels as do carbohydrates. Carbohydrates that break down rapidly to supply the body with glucose are at the high end of the index, and those that take longer to break down and digest are at the low end. Some people make the mistake of thinking that only simple carbohydrates are at the high end when, in fact, some complex carbohydrates are also at the

TABLE 2-5	Glycemic Index (GI) of Foods	
Low GI	**Medium GI**	**High GI**
Apples	Beets	Popcorn
Carrots	Cantaloupe	Watermelon
Grapes	Pineapple	Whole wheat bread
Kidney beans	Table sugar	While flour and bread
Peanuts	White and wild rice	Corn flakes
Lentils	Sweet potatoes	Cheerios
Corn	New potatoes	Baked potatoes

high end. The lower the glycemic index (GI), the less demand for insulin and slower the digestion and absorption rates. The less the demand for insulin, the better blood glucose control. People who are diabetic need to learn the glycemic value of foods in order to prepare meals that will allow for slower release of glucose into the blood stream. Table 2-5 gives a few examples of GI for foods.

PROBLEMS ASSOCIATED WITH CARBOHYDRATES

Lactose intolerance, also referred to as "milk allergy," occurs when there is an absence of the digestive enzyme lactase. Without lactase, the disaccharide lactose cannot be digested or absorbed. It passes undigested to the colon, where bacteria feed on the carbohydrate, resulting in cramping and diarrhea. People who are lactose intolerant must avoid dairy products or take lactase enzyme pills before consuming dairy products. Food for Thought 2-7 explains how lactose-intolerant people can get their daily requirement of calcium.

🍎 FOOD FOR THOUGHT 2-7

Lactose-intolerant people can substitute fruit juices fortified with highly absorbable calcium citrate, or take calcium supplements to supply the body with the daily requirement of calcium.

Certain ethnic groups are more prone to lactose intolerance: Asians, Native Americans, African Americans

- Excessive fiber intake can decrease mineral absorption and cause cramping and gas. Be sure to increase fiber in the diet gradually and drink plenty of water.
- Causes dental caries—simple sugars are most cariogenic. (See Chapter 9.)
- Excess consumption of simple CHO can cause a temporary elevation in blood triglycerides, which can increase risk for heart disease.
- Simple sugar load can cause blood glucose to spike and then drop below normal, causing "rebound" hypoglycemia.

SUGAR AS A PRESERVATIVE

Sugar is present in a wide array of processed foods, for example, cereal, canned food products, candy, and baked foods. Like salt, it can be used as a natural preservative because it pulls water from cells and disables bacteria. Most of the time, its taste is undetectable, as in canned goods, crackers, and processed foods.

CARBOHYDRATES ARE PROTEIN SPARING

Carbohydrates are called "protein sparing." The function of protein in the body is varied, but includes important tasks like creating antibodies, hormones, and building and repairing body tissue. (See Chapter 3.) When the liver stores are depleted of glucose and carbohydrate consumption is restricted, the body will build glucose from amino acids found in protein through a process called "glucogenesis."

CARBOHYDRATE RESTRICTION

Carbohydrates are needed for many metabolic functions. If a diet restricts intake of carbohydrates (low carb), there is minimal glucose available for the body to use for vital processes. If there is not enough glucose to perform vital metabolic functions, the liver will convert fat into fatty acids using adipose cells (fat cells). The rapid release of all these fatty acids creates incomplete breakdown in the liver leading to formation of ketones. Glucose is the preferred energy source for all body cells and ketones are the body's crisis reaction to lack of carbohydrates. With ketones circulating, the body enters a physiologic state of **ketosis** which is a response to fuel shortage (see Food for Thought 2-8). Because our brain and heart need a steady supply of carbohydrates for proper functioning, a state of starvation will kick the body into "survival mode," at which time it will use ketones for energy and brain and heart activity.

🍎 FOOD FOR THOUGHT 2-8

ACETONE BREATH SMELL

Acetyl groups are also made during the production of ketones which will give breath a distinctive acetone smell (fruity chemical odor).

COUNSELING PATIENTS

When providing nutritional counseling for a patient and his or her diet diary reveals a deficiency in the food groups that supply the most carbohydrates (breads and cereals, dairy, and fruits and vegetables), encourage choosing and eating more complex versus simple carbohydrates. Some patients have difficulty making sudden switches or find that the more fibrous versions of bread, rice, etc. are less palatable. Suggest mixing simple and complex carbohydrates and gradually increasing the proportion of complex carbohydrates until they are able to make the change to healthier complex versions.

For example, you can suggest that patients:

- Mix a few tablespoons of brown rice with white rice.
- Mix whole wheat pasta with semolina pasta.
- When preparing a sandwich, use one piece of white and one piece of whole grain bread, putting the white bread tongue side. Try the same with hamburger buns, rolls, and crackers.
- To increase the servings of fruits and vegetables, drink juice instead of soda.
- Add variety to meals with soft cooked and fresh vegetables.

Putting This Into Practice

Your patient has rampant facial caries on her six maxillary anterior teeth. She states that she has a problem staying awake for her job as a bank security guard on the night shift. To stay alert, she drinks a soda every other hour.

1. Would you consider the soda to be a simple sugar or a complex carbohydrate?
2. Give an explanation of what is happening in your patient's body to cause the cycle of low and high energy.
3. Suggest a drink substitution that would give her blood sugar homeostasis.
4. Evaluate your food and drink consumption over the last 2 days and determine if your intake of simple sugars was less than 20% of the total calories in your diet.
5. What changes can you make to better maintain your blood sugar level?

WEB RESOURCES

Sugar Content of Selected Foods
   http://www.nal.usda.gov/fnic/foodcomp/Data/Classics/index.html

American Society for Nutritional Sciences: Current and Archived Editions of *Journal of Nutrition* http://www.nutrition.org

Consumer Fact Sheet: Sugar in Your Diet http://www.sbreb.org/brochures/FactSheet/

Current Knowledge of the Effects of Sugar Intake
   http://www.ussugar.com/sugarnews/industry/health_effects.html

Tufts Nutrition Navigator: A Rating Guide to Nutrition Websites
   http://navigator.tufts.edu/general

The Diabetes Food Pyramid http://www.diabetes.org/nutrition-and-recipes/nutrition/sugar.jsp

Sugar Sweet by Nature http://www.sugar.org/consumers/sweet_by_nature.asp?id=279

SUGGESTED READING

van Dam RM, Seidell JC. Carbohydrate intake and obesity. *Eur. J. Clin. Nutr.* 2007; 61(Suppl 1):S75–S99.

Johnson R, Frary C. Choose beverages and foods to moderate your intake of sugars: the 2000 Dietary Guidelines for Americans—what's all the fuss about? *American Society for Nutritional Sciences Special Supplement, Symposium: Carbohydrates—Friend or Foe*, 2000.

Nappo-Dattoma L. *Carbohydrates their impact on the body and your patients' oral health by Luisa*. Access December 2006:59–61.

Simin L, Willett WC, Manson JE, et al. Relation between changes in intakes of dietary fiber and grain products and changes in weight and development of obesity among middle-aged women. *Am. J. Clin. Nutr.* 2003;78(5):920–927.

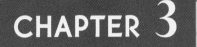

CHAPTER 3

PROTEIN

OBJECTIVES

Upon completion of this chapter, the reader will be able to:

1 Discuss the benefits of protein in the diet
2 Describe the difference between structural and functional protein and list examples of each
3 Identify essential, nonessential, and semiessential amino acids from a list
4 Explain the difference between dipeptide, tripeptide, and polypeptide bonds
5 Differentiate between complete and incomplete protein, complementary and supplementary protein
6 Identify four types of vegetarians and state foods eliminated from each type's diet
7 Outline the digestion of proteins
8 Discuss disadvantages of protein deficiency and excess and explain their effect on the body
9 Define biologic value and give examples of foods with high value
10 Discuss nitrogen balance and state situations when the body would be in positive or negative balance
11 Compute the daily Recommended Dietary Intake (RDI) of protein
12 Counsel patients on changes in the diet when they do not meet the RDI requirements

Proteins AT A GLANCE

Molecular Structure	Primary Role in Body	Source in Diet	Recommended Dietary Intake	Digestion/Absorption	Kcal/gm
COOH (carboxyl group) NH$_2$ (amino radical) Carbon and hydrogen side groups	GMR Growth Maintenance (enzymes, antibodies) Repair	Meat Dairy	40–65 g/d Depends on weight	Begins in stomach when mixed with pepsin, passes to small intestines where it mixes with trypsin and chymotrypsin, then passes through the wall and is absorbed by body; liver controls ratio of amino acids in the blood stream	4

KEY TERMS

Amino Acid
Biologic Value
Complementary Protein
Complete Protein
Dipeptide
Essential Amino Acids
    (EAAs)

Fruitarian
Incomplete Protein
Kwashiorkor
Lacto-Ovo Vegetarian
Lactovegetarian
Marasmus
Negative Nitrogen Balance

Nonessential Amino Acids
Peptide Bond
Polypeptide
Positive Nitrogen Balance
Supplementary Protein
Tripeptide
Vegan

Protein is vital for life and second only to water as the most important nutrient. Without protein we would not have muscle structure, and since muscle is what causes contractions that pump oxygen and nutrients throughout the body, we would not be able to breathe or survive. Proteins, carbohydrates, and lipids are *similar* in composition as all three contain the elements carbon, hydrogen, and oxygen, but protein *differs* from them in that it has the added element of nitrogen. Unlike carbohydrates and lipids, protein is not identifiable as a single molecule but is made up of several amino acids. Nitrogen, the differing element, is part of the amino acid "building blocks" of protein. There can be thousands of arrangements of amino acids making protein, with each arrangement doing something different for the body.

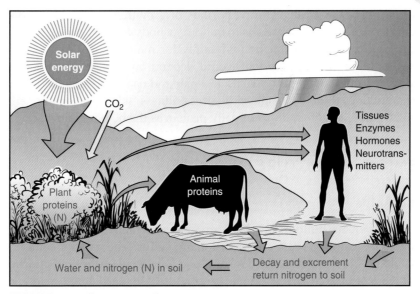

FIGURE 3-1   Proteins in the ecosystem.

NITROGEN IN THE ECOSYSTEM

Figure 3-1 illustrates how nitrogen ends up in our food and is outlined below:

1. Nitrogen is constantly cycling through the earth's ecosystem and is absorbed from the air into the soil.
2. Plants absorb nitrogen from the soil and make amino acids by combining nitrogen absorbed from the ground with carbon fragments produced during photosynthesis.
3. Plants link amino acids together to form plant proteins.
4. Animals consume plant proteins, which convert to animal protein.
5. Animal waste returns nitrogen to the soil.
6. Humans consume plant proteins directly or indirectly while eating animal products.

PRIMARY ROLE OF PROTEIN IN THE BODY

The primary role of protein in the body is for growth, maintenance, and repair. Growth is the major metabolic function of protein during youth, with children requiring more than adults. During periods of growth, a body will need larger amounts of protein on a daily basis to build new body tissues and cells.

In maturity, protein's function is mainly for maintenance. As an adult, the amount required by an individual would depend on how much protein is lost each day in urine, feces, sweat, mucus, lost hair and nails, and sloughed skin cells. Persons under high levels of physical stress, illness, injury, or emotional stress may also require larger amounts of daily protein as the body repairs itself.

CHEMICAL STRUCTURE OF PROTEIN

Amino Acids

Amino acids are the building blocks of protein that contain the elements of carbon, hydrogen, oxygen, nitrogen, and occasionally sulfur. The general configuration is: one amino group, one acid group, and one functional group that attaches to a central atom of carbon. The functional group differs for each amino acid.

1. Amino radical group—one nitrogen atom and two hydrogen atoms: NH_2.
2. Carboxyl group—one carbon atom, two oxygen atoms, and one hydrogen atom: COOH.
3. Functional group that takes the place of one of the two hydrogens off the central carbon atom. The functional group is depicted as "R" in the pictorial graphic of amino acids and is what makes each amino acid unique and distinctive.

A protein molecule is large and usually made up of more than 100 amino acids linked together. There are 20 common amino acids that can join together to form a protein molecule useful to the body. In order for amino acids to join together, two hydrogen and one oxygen are dropped (water molecule) forming a bond called a **peptide bond**. When two amino acids link together the resulting structure is called a **dipeptide** and when three are linked it is called a **tripeptide**. When there are several hundred amino acids linked together, they form a **polypeptide**. These structures can form long strands (structural protein) or a three-dimensional shape (functional protein). If you think of amino acids as jewelry beads that form bracelets, the arrangement for putting the beads together is endless.

🍎 FOOD FOR THOUGHT 3-1

Hydrolysis is a process where a single water molecule is placed between two amino acids that are bonded together.

TABLE 3-1 Essential, Nonessential, and Semiessential Amino Acids		
Essential	**Nonessential**	**Semiessential**
Isoleucine	Alanine	Cysteine[a]
Leucine	Aspartate	Tyrosine
Lysine	Asparagine	Histidine
Methionine[a]	Glutamate	Arginine
Phenylalanine	Glutamine	
Threonine	Glycine	
Tryptophan	Proline	
Valine	Serine	

[a]Contain sulfur.

Essential versus Nonessential Amino Acids

Amino acids can be either essential or nonessential. **Essential amino acids** are those which the body cannot synthesize from other compounds so they must be obtained from food. However, the body can form **nonessential amino acids** from nitrogen and a carbon chain or from a similar essential acid. Four amino acids can be considered semiessential during childhood because the metabolic pathways that synthesize these amino acids are not fully developed. The amounts required by the body depend on age and health, so it is difficult to make a general statement about dietary requirement. (See Table 3-1 for a list of essential, nonessential, and semiessential amino acids.)

Protein provides the body with many structural and functional processes and it is the *shape* of the amino acid that determines how the body uses it (Figure 3-2).

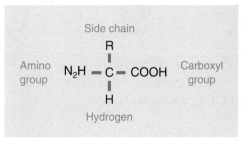

FIGURE 3-2 Amino acid chemical structure.

Structural proteins (growth)

The structure of your body today is not the structure of your body tomorrow as we are constantly degrading and making new cells and tissue. Lost hair, dry skin sloughing off, sweat, excretions, and the flip side of new hair and nail growth are just a few examples. During periods of growth, the body will wake to a new morning with more bone and muscle tissue than when it fell asleep. Protein of good quality (containing all EAAs) is needed to assist our bodies to make its complex structural parts.

- Skin
- Tendons
- Bone matrix

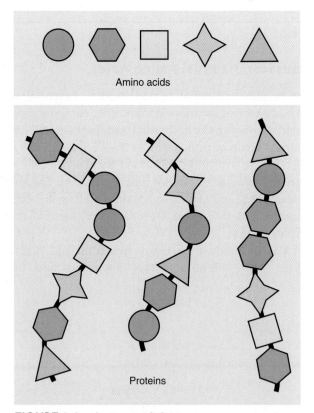

FIGURE 3-3   Amino acid shapes.

- Cartilage
- Connective tissue
- Teeth
- Eye lens

Functional proteins (maintenance and repair)

Functional proteins do not follow the same design as structural protein strands so they are more invisible and can dissolve in body fluids to be carried to all parts of the body to do their work. The amino acid chains twist and fold into a globular shape (Figure 3-3) and do the following in the body:

- Regulate activity within the body's fluid compartments
- Synthesis of hormones, enzymes, antibodies, transport proteins (lipoproteins), and chemical messengers (neurotransmitters)
- Regulates pH of the mouth

PROTEIN QUANTITY AND QUALITY

The body absorbs nitrogen from protein in the diet and can be measured to determine the quantity present in the body at any given time. There are three states of nitrogen measurement and all of us move from one state to another depending on our current situation; we can have a balanced amount of nitrogen or have more or less than our body needs. It is ideal for the body to be in nitrogen balance. Certain situations will cause the body to be in either positive nitrogen balance or negative nitrogen balance, both of which should be temporary conditions.

🍎 FOOD FOR THOUGHT 3-2

NITROGEN BALANCE

The amount of N entering the body is equal to the amount the cells need to replace parts.

- Nitrogen in = food
- Nitrogen out = urea, feces, sweat, mucus, sloughed skin, lost hair, lost nails

---

Positive nitrogen balance occurs when there is more nitrogen being absorbed and accumulated in the body than going out. This happens during periods of growth, pregnancy, muscle building, and repair of tissue after illness or injury. **Negative nitrogen balance** occurs when there is more nitrogen going out of the body than staying in, signifying loss of body protein. This state occurs during rapid weight loss, illness, fever, starvation, prolonged metabolic or emotional stress, and protein-deficient diets.

🍎 FOOD FOR THOUGHT 3-3

POSITIVE NITROGEN BALANCE

Process occurs during periods of growth, pregnancy, muscle building, and repair of tissue after injury.

🍎 FOOD FOR THOUGHT 3-4

NEGATIVE NITROGEN BALANCE

Process occurs during rapid weight loss, illness, fever, starvation, prolonged metabolic or emotional stress, and protein deficient diets.

Protein quality is determined by the combination of EAAs in a single source of food. The more EAAs in its contents, the closer it is to a perfect protein, and the more useful it is to the body. Protein-rich foods have a **biologic value** based on a grading scale of 1 to 100 (see Table 3-2 for some examples). The number it receives indicates how well nutrients from the food can be made into body protein. Foods that are closest to the value of 100 are animal-derived proteins like eggs, meat, fish, poultry, and dairy. Although plant-derived proteins are lower in fat and digest more quickly than animal sources, they do not have all the amino acids needed to form a complete protein. But just because a food does not have a high biologic value it does not mean that it should be avoided in the diet. Meal planners can be creative to combine foods that together will contain all the EAAs needed to form protein.

Complete proteins contain all the EAAs in the needed proportions. Animal protein provides complete proteins; plant protein provides incomplete protein (See Table 3-3).

Incomplete proteins are low in one or more of the EAAs.

TABLE 3-2	Estimated Biologic Value in Foods of Animal and Plant Origin
Source	**Estimated Biologic Value**
Animal Source	
Whole egg	100
Egg white	88
Cheese	84
Poultry	79
Fish	70
Lean red meat	69
Milk	60
Plant Source	
Brown rice	57
White rice	56
Peanuts	55
Peas	55
Corn	36
Potato	34

Complementary proteins form an amino acid pattern equal to that found in a complete protein by combining two foods in the same meal. An example would be combining grains and legumes; eaten together, they form a complete protein.

Supplementary protein is a small amount of a high-quality protein added to a meal that is otherwise marginal in terms of protein quantity. An example would be to add eggs, cheese, or milk to a high-carbohydrate meal.

It was once thought that for the body to utilize complementary or supplemental protein, both had to be consumed together in the same meal. Research has since

TABLE 3-3	Major Food Sources of Protein
Animal Sources	**Plant Sources**
Meat	Legumes
Milk	Peas
Eggs	Beans
Fish	Grains
Crustaceans	

revealed that the body can utilize foods that have been eaten within a few hours of each other to form complete proteins.

RECOMMENDED DIETARY INTAKE

The RDI of protein is dependent on an individual's body size and physical activity and is estimated to be 40 to 65 g/day. The standard would be at the lower end for a slightly built, sedentary person and upper end for a person with a large frame with high activity level. The amount is calculated as 0.8 g of protein/kg of body weight/day. Example:

weight of 120 lb = 55 kg
0.8 × 55 = 44 g

The daily reference value (DRV) of protein for a person weighing 120 lb is 44 g/day.

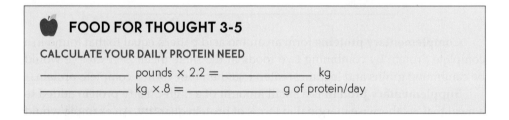

FOOD FOR THOUGHT 3-5

CALCULATE YOUR DAILY PROTEIN NEED

_____ pounds × 2.2 = _____ kg
_____ kg ×.8 = _____ g of protein/day

DIGESTION OF PROTEINS

Particles of protein-rich food are broken down to smaller pieces by chewing and grinding but the enzymes secreted in the mouth do not affect the molecular structure. After the bolus of food is swallowed and deposited in the stomach, digestion of protein begins when hydrochloric acid and pepsin (a protease) react and break apart the molecules. When the mass of partially digested food passes into the small intestine (duodenum), trypsin and chymotrypsin continue to break down the protein into a single amino acid through a process called *hydrolysis* so that it can pass through intestinal villi cells to be absorbed by the body and carried by blood to the liver. Liver cells use amino acids for protein synthesis or remove the amine group to use the carbon chain for fuel.

🍎 **FOOD FOR THOUGHT 3-6**

Pepsin is the only protease that can digest collagen.

PROTEIN DEFICIENCY

Protein deficiency occurs when the diet is lacking in this nutrient. Protein deficiency symptoms are seen in tissues that are replaced most often—red blood cells and cells lining the digestive tract. Changes that occur in the body because of protein deficiency are as follows:

- Anemia
- Lowered resistance to infection
- Edema
- Brittle and slow-growing hair and nails
- Scaly appearance to skin, with sores that will not heal

Our American diet supplies more than enough protein, so deficiencies are rare but they are still documented in developing countries. The two most documented deficiencies are:

1. **Kwashiorkor**—lack of dietary protein; edema accounts for the pot-bellied look on starving kids in undeveloped countries
2. **Marasmus**—near or total starvation from lack of calories, as in anorexia nervosa

PROTEIN EXCESS

How many times have you driven by a restaurant marquee advertising "all you can eat" or a "16-oz steak" on special? Unfortunately, the concept of protein excess is very common in most of our developed nations, sometimes to a gross extreme. My Pyramid recommends no more than 6 oz of protein-rich food source or less per day. If a diet contains more protein than the daily requirement, the body has two choices in what to do with any excess: use it for energy or store it as fat.

What happens when the body ingests more protein than it requires?

- Metabolic process dismantles protein into amino acids.
- Amino acids are metabolized, releasing energy and nitrogen.
- If the energy supply exceeds demand, the excess carbons are synthesized into fat and stored in adipose tissue.
- Excess nitrogen in the blood is processed through the liver and kidneys.
- Kidneys and liver work overtime to rid the body of excess nitrogen.

PROTEIN SUPPLEMENTS

Body builders are the number one group supporting sales of protein supplements. Protein is needed for building and maintaining muscles or repairing them from heavy workouts. But our bodies also need protein to make hormones, antibodies, and red blood cells to boost our immune system and to keep our hair, nails, and skin healthy. We cannot drink a protein supplement and tell our bodies to make or enlarge muscle mass. Our bodies will take the amino acids and put them together to build the tissue our bodies need most. Whatever is left gets excreted. Most people, including body builders, get enough protein through their diet and do not require protein supplements. Athletes' protein needs will vary depending on whether they are growing, building muscle, dieting, or training for competition. Their protein needs are higher because the recommended allowance is based on the needs of people who do not exercise. The amino acids are usually used for energy during intense exercise, especially in the absence of carbohydrates.

PROCESSED AND GRILLED MEAT HEALTH CONCERNS

Salt and nitrates are used to cure and preserve meat (lunchmeat, ham, bacon, hot dogs, salami, etc.), and both have detrimental effects on health. Excessive salt can have a direct relationship on increased incidence of high blood pressure, and nitrates used to cure meat are converted into cancer-causing nitrosamines in the stomach. For these reasons, it is wise to limit processed meat in the diet. Including foods rich in vitamin C, such as tomatoes and orange juice, with the meal can prevent the conversion of nitrates to nitrosamines.

When using a cooking method with muscle meat, poultry, or fish that results in charring or blackening (e.g., barbecuing or grilling), fat drips onto the coals, forming a smoke that penetrates the meat. The effect of smoke penetrating the meat forms heterocyclic amines and polycyclic aromatic hydrocarbons—both of which are cancer-causing chemicals. It is recommended that lean cuts of meat be used when grilling and to limit foods prepared this way.

VEGETARIANISM

Many famous people were vegetarians: Socrates, Leonardo da Vinci, Benjamin Franklin, Mahatma Gandhi, Albert Einstein, and Clara Barton, just to name a few. The American Institute for Cancer Research has recently reported that close to 40% of teens identify themselves as vegetarians, and it is estimated that close to 5 million Americans have elected to eliminate meat, poultry, and fish from their diets. Reasons for choosing this eating pattern are varied and include health, religion, ethics, weight, fashion, and environment. The American Dietetic Association has published a new food guide that outlines how to choose a meatless diet but still consume all the needed nutrients. Diets rich in vegetables, fruits, leafy greens, whole grains, nuts and seeds, and legumes can meet the protein needs of people from all age-groups and all walks of life.

When meat is excluded from a diet, it leaves room for more carbohydrates, and oftentimes plant sources of protein are forgotten. The type of carbohydrates substituted matters, because eating more simple sugars opens the door for increased incidence of caries and diseases. Vegetarians should choose foods wisely and include complex carbohydrates to ensure that there is enough protein in the diet. In the United States, vegan diets are usually lower in protein than the standard diet; however, the recommendations are very generous and diets high in protein do not appear to have any health advantages. (Protein is needed in very small quantities, approximately 1 out of every 10 calories.) There are several types of vegetarians, depending on what they include in their diets:

- **Lacto-ovo vegetarian**—includes eggs and dairy products with meals
- **Lactovegetarian**—dairy products are only foods of animal origin
- **Vegan**—consumes no foods of animal origin
- **Fruitarian**—eats only fruits

🍎 FOOD FOR THOUGHT 3-7

Which type of vegetarian would have the least trouble obtaining protein in his or her diet?

Meatless foods that can serve as good protein sources are:

- Beans
- Nuts
- Seeds

- Tofu
- Soy foods
- Vegetarian meat substitutes
- Eggs
- Dairy products

Completely eliminating animal protein from the diet can create a deficiency in *vitamin B₁₂*, which is found only in animal foods. The deficiency develops over time, affecting the central nervous system, and is not manifested until after the body's stores are depleted, usually 4 years' worth. Once the deficiency manifests, it is irreversible. Lacto-ovo vegetarians need not worry, because B₁₂ is supplied in cow's milk. A true vegan, however, must supplement his or her diet with fortified soy milk or meat replacement.

🍎 FOOD FOR THOUGHT 3-8

Some of the symptoms of vitamin B_{12} deficiency are anemia, fatigue, constipation, anorexia, weight loss, numbness and tingling of hands and feet, depression, confusion, poor memory, and soreness of the mouth and tongue.

DISADVANTAGES OF VEGETARIANISM

Lack of animal foods can cause deficiencies in:

- Vitamin B₁₂ (can take as a supplement)
- Vitamin D (need exposure to the sun)
- Iron (plant iron is not as absorbable as animal iron)
- Calcium and riboflavin (can be obtained in soy products)

🍎 FOOD FOR THOUGHT 3-9

Meeting calcium needs can be accomplished by including soy milk, soy nuts, fortified fruit juices, fortified cereal, and calcium-rich vegetables such as broccoli, kale, and bok choy. Spinach is also high in calcium, but the oxalate binds with the calcium, reducing its absorption.

BENEFITS OF VEGETARIANISM

- Usually maintains desired weight for height
- Lower blood cholesterol
- Lower rates of some forms of cancer
- Better digestive function
- Benefits the earth

🍎 FOOD FOR THOUGHT 3-10

ADVANTAGES OF VEGETARIANISM

Plant proteins are:
- Higher in fiber than meats
- Richer in certain vitamins and minerals
- Lower in fat

🍎 FOOD FOR THOUGHT 3-11

ECOLOGICAL THOUGHT

It takes 17 acres of grazing land to produce 1 million calories of animal protein, but one well-developed acre of plants can raise 1 million calories of plant-based protein.

COUNSELING PATIENTS

Most people report more than adequate servings for the meat group because of its abundance in our American diet. If your client reports more servings than suggested for this food group, advise as to what constitutes a serving size. The proper portion size for meat will be the same as a deck of cards, a box of jello, or small digital camera. Many people are unaware that restaurant serving sizes are grossly oversized. If the patient is deficient in the meat group, the following suggestions can be made:

- Hard-boil eggs and store them in the refrigerator to add to salads and sandwiches.

- Include cheese, eggs, nuts, and beans with salads.
- Cook a 12-oz steak for dinner, but save half for a sandwich or casserole the next day.
- Include more poultry and fish and less red or fatty meat.
- Educate as to sources of alternative protein—milk, beans, cheese, nuts, and so on.
- If your client is eating hot dogs or other processed meats, remind him or her to consume them with vitamin C to offset harmful effects of nitrosamines.
- Suggest two meatless dinners each week.
- Encourage meal preparation using chopped chicken, turkey, or beef with pasta or rice, versus large servings of each.

Putting This Into Practice

Your patient is a 19-year-old college student who has made the decision to eliminate animal food products from her diet.

1. Write your explanation of the dangers of substituting carbohydrate-rich foods for the calories lost from eliminating protein-rich foods.
2. Calculate her daily protein needs based on a body weight of 126 lb.
3. List foods that can be included in her diet to ensure an adequate daily protein intake.
4. Write your explanation of how inadequate protein intake can affect the oral cavity.

WEB RESOURCES

Harvard: Protein Moving Closer to Center Stage
http://www.hsph.harvard.edu/nutritionsource/protein.html
Atkins Diet and Low Carbohydrate Support (Canada) http://www.lowcarb.ca
Atkins Nutritionals http://atkins.com
Beyond Vegetarianism—Transcending Outdated Dogmas http://www.beyondveg.com
International Vegetarian Union http://www.ivu.org

The Linus Pauling Institute—Nitrosamines and Cancer
    http://lpi.oregonstate.edu/f-w00/nitrosamine.html

MedlinePlus Medical Encyclopedia—Protein in Diet
    http://www.nlm.nih.gov/medlineplus/ency/article/002467.htm

Newswise—Safer Outdoor Grilling Guidelines, Reducing Cancer Risk
    http://www.newswise.com/articles/view/?id=GRILL.OHM

Purdue University Animal Sciences—Meat Quality and Safety/Reduce Your Cancer Risk
    from Grilled Meat http://ag.ansc.purdue.edu/meat_quality/grilling.html

The Vegetarian Resource Group: Protein in the Vegan Diet

http://www.vrg.org/nutrition/protein.htm

SUGGESTED READING

American Dietetic Association, Dietitians of Canada. Position of the American Dietetic Association and Dietitians of Canada: vegetarian diets. *J Am Diet Assoc.* 2003;103(6):748–765.
Liebman B. The truth about the Atkins diet. *Nutr Action* 2002;29:3–7.
Mangels R. The Vegetarian Resource Group. *Protein in the vegan diet.* Available at: http://www.vrg.org/. Accessed June 2003.

CHAPTER 4

LIPIDS

OBJECTIVES

Upon completion of the chapter, the reader will be able to:

1 Name the chemical components of lipids

2 List the primary role of lipids in the diet and give examples of benefits to the body

3 State the three major categories of lipids

4 Differentiate between unsaturated fatty acid and saturated fatty acid (SFA) and choose which is healthier for the body

5 Explain the nature of fats and oils that have single and double bonds

6 Give examples of monounsaturated and polyunsaturated oils

7 Identify two essential fatty acids (EFAs) and list foods in which they are found

8 Explain the process of hydrogenation and its relationship to trans fats

9 Explain the necessity for phospholipids

10 Name three common sterols and their relationship to cardiovascular disease

11 Outline the process of lipid digestion and explain the participation of chylomicrons in the digestive process

12 State the dietary reference value (DRV) for lipids in the diet, differentiating levels for saturated and unsaturated fats

Lipids AT A GLANCE

Molecular Structure	Primary Role in Body	Source in Diet	Recommended Dietary Intake	Digestion/Absorption	Kcal/g
Carbon atom with a carboxyl end (COOH) and methyl end (CH₃)	Insulates against cold Cushion organs Energy Cell structure Provides fat-soluble vitamins	Butter, oil Marbleized meat Dairy products Sauces and salad dressing	<30% of total daily calories consumed	Begins in mouth when mixed with lipase and continues in stomach when mixed with gastric lipase. Emulsified by bile and pancreatic lipase in small intestines. Passes through wall of small intestines where absorbed by body	9

KEY TERMS

Chylomicron

Essential Fatty Acid

Fatty Acid

High-Density Lipoprotein (HDL)

Hydrogenation

Lipoprotein

Low-Density Lipoprotein (LDL)

Monounsaturated

Partially Hydrogenated

Phospholipid

Polyunsaturated

Saturated

Sterol

Trans Fat

Triglyceride

Very Low-Density Lipoprotein (VLDL)

The broad category of lipids includes oils and fats, although the word "lipid" is often used interchangeably with "fat." Lipids are an important major nutrient supplied by our diets and used for many purposes in our bodies. Chemically, lipids contain carbon, hydrogen, oxygen, and sometimes phosphorous. They have the unique general characteristic of being insoluble in water. In solution, lipids will either float or roll around in globules. Imagine mixing cooking oil or a pat of butter in a glass of water.

Intake of dietary fat has received a lot of public attention and is of special concern to those wishing to maintain a healthy body image. It is common knowledge that the fat we consume can be stored in the body and the more fat stored, the larger our pant size. But "fat" may not necessarily deserve its universal bad reputation. The right kind of fat, when eaten in moderation, has value in both the diet and body.

PRIMARY ROLE OF LIPIDS IN THE BODY

Lipids function in the body in the following important ways:

- Insulate against the cold
- Cushion organs against injury
- Are components of every body cell
- Are a good source of energy
- Give a sense of satiety and slow digestion
- Carry fat-soluble vitamins A, D, E, and K
- Make food taste good and give it a preferred smooth and creamy texture

TRIGLYCERIDES

Triglycerides are the largest category of lipids, comprising 95% of all fats found in food and body adipose tissue (fat depot). When stored in adipose tissue, they become the body's largest fuel reserve and provide vital insulation. Having fat stored in adipose cells is like having your own utility company to draw from during an energy crisis. And when it accumulates subcutaneously, it can act as a blanket that insulates against the cold or a shock absorber to cushion delicate organs such as the kidneys.

Triglyceride molecules contain carbon, oxygen, and hydrogen atoms arranged in two parts: the foundation molecule is *glycerol* and there are three *fatty acid* chains off the side. The fatty acid chains consist of carbon atoms with attached hydrogen and oxygen (COOH) (Figure 4-1).

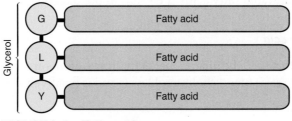

FIGURE 4-1   Fatty acid.

Fatty Acids

Triglycerides differ in their fatty acid composition, the difference being the number of carbon atoms in their chains and the number of double bonds. Fatty acid carbon chains can be short, medium, or long:

- Short—four or less carbons (short chains mix better in water—like milk)
- Medium—5 to 10 carbons
- Long—more than 12 carbons

Saturation of Fatty Acids

Fatty acids can be categorized as saturated, monounsaturated, or polyunsaturated, depending on how the carbon atoms are bonded together and whether they have a single or double bond. When a triglyceride is saturated it means all carbon atoms have bonded to hydrogen (single bond) and there are no carbon atoms joining with the carbon next to it (double bond). When one carbon in the chain joins with another, it has a double bond and is called "monounsaturated fat." If there is more than one place along the chain where a carbon bonds with another, it will have many double bonds and is called a "polyunsaturated fat."

Single bonds between carbon and hydrogen result in a straight flexible chain that will pack into a hard fat such as lard, butter, and stick margarine. Think of toy blocks stacking neatly. Double bonds between carbons result in a bend at the site of the double bond. This bend does not allow the lipid to pack neatly, so it stays liquid at room temperature, like cooking oil. Think of several random toys thrown into a bag, unable to stack together. The more double bonds a fatty acid has, the softer the fat is at room temperature.

The saturation of fatty acids is as follows and is illustrated in Figure 4-2:

- **Saturated fatty acids** (SFAs)—no double bonds
- **Monounsaturated fatty acids** (MUFAs)—one double bond
- **Polyunsaturated fatty acids** (PUFAs)—more than one double bond

Saturated fatty acid

Carbon chains that hold the full number of hydrogen atoms are said to be saturated. An SFA tends to raise blood cholesterol levels and is positively correlated with the following:

- Increased risk of cardiovascular disease
- Hypertension
- Colon cancer

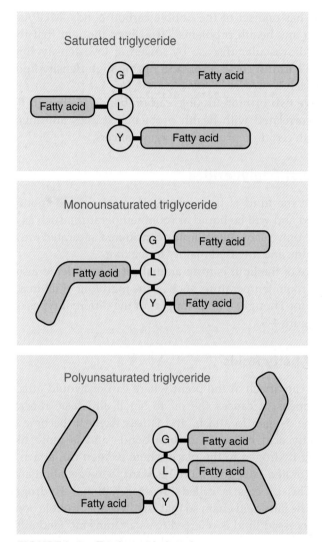

FIGURE 4-2   **Triglyceride bond.**

Unsaturated fatty acid

Carbons that hold less than the maximum number of hydrogen atoms will double bond with themselves. (Carbon bonds with another carbon.) Two common unsaturated fatty acids are as follows:

1. Monounsaturated (oleic acid)
2. Polyunsaturated (linoleic acid)

An MUFA has one set of the double carbon bonds. MUFAs have not been associated with any health problems.[1] It is even thought that they may reduce the risk of cardiovascular disease by lowering low-density lipoprotein (LDL) cholesterol, the harmful cholesterol, and raising high-density lipoprotein (HDL), the good cholesterol.

PUFAs have two or more double carbon bonds. Although PUFAs have not been directly correlated with health problems, studies are ongoing as to their relationship with certain reproductive organ cancers.

Food Source of Triglycerides

If the source of the lipid is from plants, it is considered monounsaturated or polyunsaturated and will be liquid at room temperature, such as olive, corn, and canola oils. The only plant source lipids considered saturated are the tropical oils coconut and palm, and are used mainly for baking.

If the source of the lipid is from animals, it is considered a saturated fat and will be solid at room temperature, such as the marbling of fat in a piece of beef or pork (see Food for Thought 4-2). Examples of the different types of fatty acids are presented in Figure 4-3.

Oxidation of Fatty Acids

Oxygen atoms can attach at the point where carbon would attach to hydrogen. When this happens, it causes the oil to smell and taste rancid. An SFA has nowhere for the oxygen to attach, and is less likely to become spoiled. But an unsaturated fatty acid has open carbon bonds and is more likely to become rancid. Infusing hydrogen to the place where oxygen can attach to carbons will make the unsaturated fatty acid more resistant to oxygenation and solid at room temperature. This process is called "hydrogenation." **Hydrogenation** infuses hydrogen into the fatty acid chain so that any "vacant" double bonds become full. This type of processed lipid is referred to as a "trans fat" and affects the body in the same way a saturated fat does. Food manufacturers use this process to make their product more spreadable, for example, changing corn oil into margarine or making oily natural peanut butter more creamy. Hydrogenation is what turns liquid oil into Crisco or stick margarines. Trans fats also make an oil more stable so that it can be reused (e.g., for deep frying).

Trans Fat

Most unsaturated fatty acids have the hydrogen atom on the same side of the double bond. This is called the "*cis* form." In the *trans form*, the hydrogen atoms are

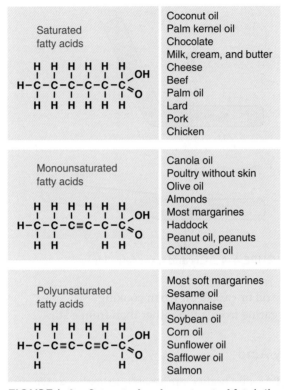

FIGURE 4-3   Saturated and unsaturated fats/oils.

on opposite sides of the double bond. This different configuration of the trans form causes the fatty acid to have a "kink." Figure 4-4 shows the difference between cis and trans oleic acids. Fatty acids that are kinked do not stack as well as those that are straight.

Trans fats are created when oils are "partially hydrogenated." Once the food product has been infused with hydrogen, it is no longer considered saturated, monounsaturated, or polyunsaturated. Up till recently, trans fats were invisible on a food label because they were excluded when computing fat calories and grams. But public concern has forced lawmakers to require that manufacturers consider trans fats in overall fat content. Now all food labels must state whether a food product contains saturated fat as well as trans fat, because even though they were hidden on the label, they were as damaging to arteries as saturated fat. Trans fats raise blood cholesterol as much as saturated fat, making it a secret killer.[2-4]

You can cut trans fats from your diet by the following:

- Avoiding foods listing "partially hydrogenated oil" as an ingredient
- Avoiding deep fried foods

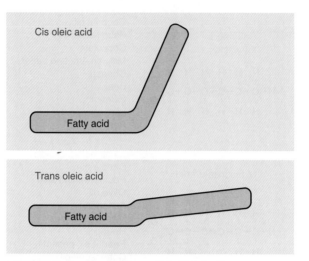

FIGURE 4-4   Cis and trans fats "kinks."

- Using olive oil or canola oil when cooking
- Using margarine from a tub rather than from a stick

Essential Fatty Acid

There are two **EFAs** our bodies are unable to make so we must get them from foods in our diets. They are commonly referred to as "omega oils":

1. Omega-3: linolenic acid; found in flaxseed, canola, or soybean oil, walnuts, tuna, and salmon
2. Omega-6: linoleic acid; found in vegetable oils

The number after omega indicates on which carbon the double bond is located. Omega-3 has been referred to as the "anticardiovascular disease nutrient." Our bodies are always forming and destroying tiny blood clots, and omega-3 helps form substances that reduce blood clot formation, thereby keeping our blood "thin."

PHOSPHOLIPIDS

Phospholipids are the second category of lipids in our food and body. Chemically, a phospholipid looks like a triglyceride except it contains a phosphorus-containing molecule attached in place of one of the fatty acids. Phospholipids function in our bodies as emulsfiers that keep molecules of fat and water in solution. They also

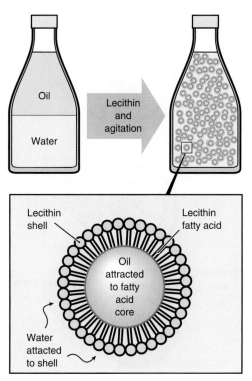

FIGURE 4-5   **Action of a phospholipid.**

make up the cell membrane and control movement of materials in and out of a cell. Phospholipids are great for cooking and baking because they can keep ingredients from separating. A common phospholipid is lecithin (Figure 4-5), which is found naturally in soybeans and egg yolks. Read the labels of food in your pantry to see which products may contain lecithin.

STEROLS

Sterols are the third category of lipids with a distinction of carbon rings instead of chains and contain no fatty acids. Cholesterol is the most well-known sterol in our food and bodies, but its benefit in our diet continues to be debated. Cholesterol is used in our bodies as a precursor to making vitamin D and sex hormones, like testosterone and progesterone. And although we need it for these necessary functions, excessive intake of cholesterol-rich foods has been associated with the development of cardiovascular disease. Routinely eating cholesterol-laden food promotes build up of fatty deposits in arteries in genetically sensitive people. Most

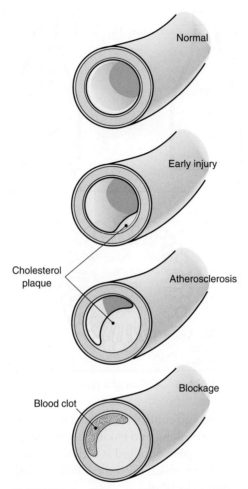

FIGURE 4-6   Stages of blocked arteries.

foods high in cholesterol are also high in saturated fats (Figure 4-6), which are more detrimental to the arteries than the cholesterol.

LIPOPROTEINS TRANSPORT LIPIDS

Because oil and water do not mix, the body has its own way of allowing fat to travel through the bloodstream to bring lipids to every body cell. **Lipoproteins** are soluble in both oil and water, so they can circulate freely through the blood. Packaged this way, fats can remain soluble and not separate from liquid blood.

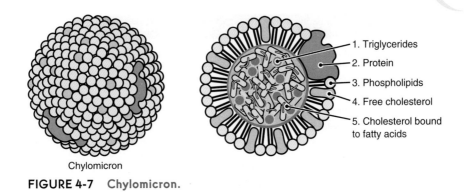

1. Triglycerides
2. Protein
3. Phospholipids
4. Free cholesterol
5. Cholesterol bound to fatty acids

Chylomicron

FIGURE 4-7   Chylomicron.

Lipoproteins are triglycerides coated with protein, cholesterol, and phospholipids. A **chylomicron** is a type of packaged lipoprotein that is formed during lipid absorption in the small intestines and transported by the lymph system into the bloodstream to be utilized by the body for energy (Figure 4-7).

🍎 FOOD FOR THOUGHT 4-1

Chylo means milky and micron means small: after eating a high-fat meal, the blood is so full of chylomicrons it appears milky.

Besides chylomicrons, there are three other types of important lipoproteins: **HDLs, LDLs, very low-density lipoproteins** (VLDLs). HDLs are made in the liver and small intestine and consist of more protein than cholesterol. LDLs, on the other hand, are denser in cholesterol than protein. LDLs carry the cholesterol to the heart's arteries, where it penetrates the vessel walls and narrows or "clogs" the arteries and restricts blood flow, giving LDL an unhealthy reputation. HDLs are considered healthy because they actually have a protective factor against LDL. HDLs can remove cholesterol from vessel walls and take it back to the liver, where it is excreted with body waste. VLDL is mostly cholesterol and very little protein, and like LDL, contributes to cardiovascular disease. VLDL transports endogenous cholesterol, whereas the HDL and LDL transport dietary cholesterol.

Food for Thought 4-2 contains a tip for remembering the difference between HDL and LDL.

Desirable blood cholesterol should be below 200 mg/dL. An average-weight person should limit daily dietary cholesterol intake to less than

TABLE 4-1	Foods that Contain Cholesterol
One Cup Food	**Cholesterol (mg)**
Ice cream	84
Egg noodles	50
Whole milk	34
Low-fat milk	20
Skim milk	5
Chicken liver	800
Beef brains	2,100
Other	
Hot dog	100
Lobster (3 oz)	100
Shrimp (3 oz)	100
Cheesecake (9 in.)	2,053

(Taken from Nutrition for Dental Hygienists by Morris and Knight.)

300 mg/day. Table 4-1 indicates the amount of cholesterol contained in certain foods.

🍎 FOOD FOR THOUGHT 4-2

TIPS FOR REMEMBERING HDL AND LDL

↑ LDL = ↓ risk of cardiovascular disease
↑HDL = ↓ risk of cardiovascular disease

Think of the H in HDL and put it in Healthy.

🍎 FOOD FOR THOUGHT 4-3

CHOLESTEROL GUIDELINES FOR THE AVERAGE AMERICAN ADULT

(http://www.mayoclinic.com/health/cholesterol-levels/cl00001)
Total cholesterol level should be less than 200.
LDL level should be less than 130.
HDL levels should be 50 to 75 or higher.

RECOMMENDED DIETARY INTAKE

On the basis of a 2,000 total daily calorie intake, it has been suggested that no more than 30% of total calories should be from fat. Only 10% should be saturated fat. Another way to figure the amount of fat in a diet is to count grams. When counting grams, there should be no more than 65 and 20 g of saturated fat. It is wise for individuals with genetic tendencies for cardiovascular disease, cancer, weight control, and autoimmune diseases such as multiple sclerosis[4–7] to reduce their recommended dietary intake even more.

🍎 FOOD FOR THOUGHT 4-4

Avocados are accused of being laden with fat. According to www.avocado.org, the fruit contributes 20 vitamins, minerals, and beneficial plant compounds. The fat content is monosaturated and polyunsaturated, which means it is healthier than saturated fat.

DIGESTION OF FATS

Fats begin their digestion in the mouth with the help of lingual lipase secreted from oral salivary glands and then with gastric lipase that gets secreted when it enters the stomach. Fat remains in the stomach longer than carbohydrates and proteins, which gives the sense of fullness for a longer period of time. Digestion continues in the small intestine (duodenum), where chyme (a mixture of food, acids, and enzymes) is emulsified by bile and further broken down by pancreatic lipase. The liver produces bile and stores it in the gall bladder until it is needed for digestion of fat. Bile enters the small intestine via the bile duct. Emulsification by bile turns fat molecules into smaller particles, making it easier for lipase to break fat molecules into fatty acids and glycerol. Short-chain and medium-chain fatty acids make their way to the liver, and the long-chain fatty acids are converted into chylomicrons and dumped into the lymph system, which carries the chylomicrons through the bloodstream. Any fatty acids not used for fuel are repackaged and stored in adipose tissues. Unabsorbed cholesterol is bound by soluble fiber and eliminated from the body. (Eating soluble fiber keeps cholesterol levels low.) The mixture of reduced fat and bile is absorbed through the small intestinal villi.

> ### 🍎 FOOD FOR THOUGHT 4-5
>
> ENVIRONMENTAL CONCERNS
>
> Plants and animals absorb fat-soluble chemicals, such as pesticides, that are stored in fat and oil. People who use these plants and animals as food will absorb some of the stored chemicals, such as dichlorodiphenyltrichloroethane (DDT).

OBESITY

Years ago, being obese signified that a person had enough money to afford the luxury of a steady diet. Currently, these same individuals would no longer be looked upon as persons of wealth and stature. Instead, they would be considered players in a growing epidemic which has proved to be detrimental to a body's health.

Gradually, over a period of many years, our diets changed from being high in complex carbohydrates to being high in simple sugars and fat. The food processing industry contributed to the change by using sugar, sodium, and hydrogenated fat to keep food from becoming spoiled and rancid. Fast food industry contributed by ramping up portion sizes to steal patrons from competing chains. In addition, improvements in technology minimized our daily movements and offered more sedentary forms of entertainment. Add these changes together and you have a recipe to produce individuals who are the walking unhealthy.

According to the World Health Organization (WHO), the cause of obesity is the direct result of excess calorie consumption with decreased expenditure of energy. Their 2003 report states that worldwide, more than 1 billion adults are overweight, with 300 million of them being clinically obese. Twenty-two million children younger than 5 years are already overweight. Obesity-related diseases include type 2 diabetes, cardiovascular disease, hypertension, stroke, and some cancers. Statistics of this magnitude explains why medical care facilities claim they are overburdened with patients seeking care for obesity-related diseases and disabilities.

> ### 🍎 FOOD FOR THOUGHT 4-6
>
> Liposuction, the process of sucking out excess fat deposits in the body, is not a treatment for obesity or substitution for healthy diet and exercise. And it is not a quick fix for cellulite that causes dimpled-looking skin on thighs and buttocks. Removing certain pockets of fat can reshape the body giving more desirable contours. According to www.plasticsurgery.org, more than 450,000 lipoplasty procedures were performed in 2007.

COUNSELING PATIENTS

When analyzing a patient's diet diary, consider if his or her food choices are high or low fat. Demonstrate how to configure 30% reference daily intake (RDI) for fat with only 10% saturated fat. Sections of MyPyramid that contain the most lipids are the dairy and meat group. Inquire if they consciously choose low-fat dairy products or choose lean cuts of meat.

The following are examples of how to encourage low-fat food selections:

- An acronym to remember is when choosing meat is FiRST, which stands for flank, round, sirloin, and tenderloin. These four cuts are considered the leanest.
- Vegetarians may choose cheese as a protein substitution. If so, they need to know that 85% to 90% of the calories in cheese come from fat, much of which is saturated.
- If your patient is drinking whole milk, a sudden switch to skim or fat-free milk may be too big of a change and result in failure. Suggest gradually switching by drinking 2% for a few weeks, then switching to 1% for a few weeks, and then eventually working down to fat-free. Sometimes mixing the two—whole and skim—works also. There is just as much calcium in skim milk as there is in whole milk.
- If your patient is using high-fat spreads, suggest trying some of the fat-free margarines and cream cheeses.
- When choosing a topping for baked potatoes and in pasta salads, fat-free salad dressings and salsa are good substitutions.
- Encourage using monounsaturated and polyunsaturated cooking oils.
- Identify food sources of EFAs—omega 3 and omega 6
- Educate about trans fats and teach your client how to spot them on food labels.
- Almost any food from the fruit and vegetable food group is fat-free. Three exceptions are olives, avocados, and coconuts.

Putting This Into Practice

Your 45-year-old female patient has recently visited a Bariatric Clinic hoping to lose at least 50 lb. She was considering gastric bypass surgery but agreed, at her doctor's suggestion, to first try prescription medication to suppress

(continued)

her appetite for 3 months. She reported taking bupropion, lipitor, and hydrochlorothiazide (HCTZ) and over-the-counter prenatal vitamins. On clinical examination, you noticed xerostomia and five new-class five carious lesions on the facial of tooth numbers 3, 4, 5, 14, and 15.

On the basis of the above information, answer the following questions:

1. What effect, if any, would each of the prescribed medications have on her oral cavity?
2. What factors contributed to the development of five new-class five carious lesions?
3. What would you expect to find after disclosing her mouth?
4. What advice and instruction would you give this patient?

Your patient is a 250-lb male who lumbers back to the operatory. He has difficulty fitting in the treatment chair and is clearly out of breath from the mild exertion of walking and sitting. He makes the comment that he has to "lose some weight" and asks if you have any advice. Keeping in mind that it is not within the realm of dental nutritional counseling to "put a patient on a diet," think about some words of wisdom you can offer this patient.

1. List diseases that are caused by excess lipid consumption.
2. How can your patient find out if a food product contains a trans fat?
3. If your patient does not want to give up the amount of food he eats, give him examples of low-fat foods that can replace high-fat foods.
4. Would you expect to see any oral changes from the consumption of foods with excess fat?

WEB RESOURCES

Center for Disease Control and Prevention. Obesity and Overweight
   http://www.cdc.gov/nccdphp/dnpa/obesity/index.htm
Mayo Clinic. Fat Grams or Percentages? Which are More Important?
   http://www.mayoclinic.com/health/fat-grams/HQ00671

Science. Insecticide Content of Diet and Body Fat of Alaskan Natives

http://www.sciencemag.org/cgi/content/abstract/134/3493/1880

Cholesterol Information Online. http://www.cholesterol-information.org/

WHO Global strategies on diet, physical activity and health

http://www.who.int/dietphysicalactivity/publications/facts/obesity/en/

REFERENCES

1. Lada AT, Rudel LL. Dietary monounsaturated versus polyunsaturated fatty acids: which is really better for protection from coronary heart disease. *Curr Opin Lipidol* 2003;14(1):41–46.
2. Food and Drug Administration, HHS. Food labeling: trans fatty acids in nutrition labeling, nutrient content claims, and health claims. Final rule. *Fed Regist* 2003;68(133): 41433–41506.
3. Steinhart H, Rickert R, Winkler K. Trans fatty acids: analysis, occurrence, intake and clinical relevance. *Eur J Med Res* 2003;8(8):358–362.
4. Clifton PM, Keogh JB, Noakes M. Trans fatty acids in adipose tissue and the food supply are associated with myocardial infarction. *J Nutr* 2004;134(4):874–879.
5. Liebman B. Fat chance—extra pounds can increase your cancer risk. *Nutr Action* 2003; 30(8):3–8.
6. Lichtenstein AH. Dietary fat and cardiovascular disease risk: quantity or quality? *J Womens' Health* 2003;12(2):109–114.
7. Hu FB, Willett WC. Optimal diets for prevention of coronary heart disease. *JAMA* 2002;288(20):2569–2578.

SUGGESTED READING

Burton S, Creyer EH, Kees J, et al. Attacking the obesity epidemic: the potential health benefits of providing nutrition information in restaurants. *Am J Public Health* 2006; 96(9):1669–1675.

Chaput J, Gilbert J, Caron C. Address the obesity epidemic: what is the dentist's role? *J Can Dent Assoc* 2007;73(8):707–709.

Drummond S. Obesity: a diet that is acceptable is more likely to succeed. *J Fam Health Care* 2007;17(6):219–221.

Duley S, Fitzpatrick P. The Bariatric Treatment Team. *Dimens Dent Hyg* 2006;4(11):14–16.

Golde M, Risbeck C. The fattening of America and its effect on oral health. *Dimens Dent Hyg* 2006;4(1):16–17,35.

Kranz S, Lin PJ, Wagstaff DA. Children's dietary intake in the United States: too little, too fat? *J Pediatr* 2007;151(6):643–646.

Nicklas T, Johnson R. Position of the American Dietetic Association: dietary guidance for healthy children ages 2 to 11 years. *J Am Diet Assoc* 2004;104(4):660–677.

Ryan-Harshman M, Aldoori W. Diet and colorectal cancer: review of the evidence. *Can Fam Physician* 2007;53(11):1913–1920.

Wang Y, Beydoun MA. The obesity epidemic in the United States—gender, age, socioeconomic, racial/ethnic, and geographic characteristics: a systematic review and meta-regression analysis. *Epidemiol Rev* 2007;29:6–28.

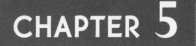

CHAPTER 5

VITAMINS

OBJECTIVES

Upon completion of the chapter, the reader will be able to:

1 Outline the discovery of vitamins
2 Identify factors that distinguish between fat-soluble and water-soluble vitamins and list vitamins in each category
3 Discuss the difference between digestion of water-soluble and fat-soluble vitamins
4 Explain how individuals can have a vitamin toxicity or imbalance
5 List precursors of the vitamins that can be synthesized by the body
6 State the four major functions of vitamins in the body
7 Using tables and charts, identify source, recommended daily intake (RDI), and excess and deficiency states of 13 vitamins

KEY TERMS

Anitoxidant	Fortification	Water Soluble
Enriched	Precursor	
Fat Soluble	Synthesis	

Vitamins AT A GLANCE

Water-Soluble Vitamins		Function	RDI	Food Sources	Deficiency	Excess	Oral Deficiency Symptoms
Thiamin	B₁	Energy metabolism	1.1 mg	Pork, fortified cereal, grains, meat, poultry, peanut butter, and eggs	Beriberi	—	—
Riboflavin	B₂	Production of ATP	1.1 mg	Milk, meat, poultry, fish, enriched whole grains, and cereals	Ariboflavinosis	—	Red swollen lips; vertical fissures; chelosis; burning, smooth red tongue; atrophied lingual papillae; red, burning gingival tissues
Niacin	B₃	Cell function Coenzyme to B₂ RBC formation	12 mg	Meat, poultry, fish, dark green leafy vegetables, enriched grains, peanut butter, and peas	Pellagra	Causes facial flushing Decreased blood lipids	—
Pyroxidine	B₆	Coenzyme in reactions for amino acid, fatty acid, and CHO metabolism	1.4 mg	Meat, poultry, fish, liver, eggs, brown rice, lentils, and peanuts	Microcytic anemia Depression Convulsions	Permanent neurologic damage Numbness in extremities Uncoordinated muscle movement	Deficiency causes angular chelitis and glossitis
Folate	B₉	Synthesize amino acids RBC maturation Synthesis of DNA and RNA	400 μg	Fortified grains, yeast, kidney, and dark green leafy vegetables	Fetal neural tube defects Macrocytic anemia	—	—
Cobalamine	B₁₂	RBC production DNA synthesis	2.4 μg	Meat, poultry, fish, eggs, and dairy	Pernicious anemia Permanent nerve and brain damage	—	—

Vitamins *AT A GLANCE (continued)*

Water-Soluble Vitamins		Function	RDI	Food Sources	Deficiency	Excess	Oral Deficiency Symptoms
Ascorbic acid	C	Collagen formation Strengthens immune system Iron and calcium absorption	60 mg	Kiwi, citrus, strawberries, cantaloupe, leafy greens, and cruciferous vegetables	Scurvy	GI upset Diarrhea Orange urine Interferes with anticoagulants Iron toxicity	Red purplish, swollen, bleeding gingival tissues Loose teeth Slow healing

Fat-Soluble Vitamins		Function	RDI	Food Sources	Deficiency	Excess	Oral Deficiency Symptoms
	A	Formation of epithelium, skin, and mucous membranes Healthy eyes Bone remodeling	800 µg	Carrots, yellow and orange fruits and vegetables, spinach, broccoli, liver, eggs, butter, and fortified foods	Hypovitaminosis A Xeropthalmia Night blindness	Headache Vomiting Double vision Hair loss Bone abnormalities Liver damage	Xerostomia Oral leukoplakia Hyperkeratosis Hyperplastic gingival tissue
	D	Absorption of calcium and phosphorus Bone formation	5–10 µg	Liver, egg yolks, and fish oil	Rickets Osteomalacia	Kidney stones Calcified blood vessels	Failure of bone wounds to heal Enamel hypocalcification Loss of alveolar bone Thinning trabeculation
	E	Antioxidant Protects RBCs	15 mg	Margarine, vegetable shortening, salad dressing, whole grains, nuts, and legumes	Hemolytic anemia	Nausea Diarrhea Cramps Interferes with anticoagulants	No known deficiency symptoms May delay clotting
	K	Synthesis for prothrombin	100 µg	Dark green leafy vegetables	Prolonged bleeding Hemorrhage	Increased clotting time	Failure of wounds to stop bleeding

RDI, recommended daily intake; ATP, adenosine triphosphate; RBC, red blood cell; GI, gastrointestinal.

"Vitamine" was the term coined by Casimir Funk (1884 to 1967) for the unidentified substances present in food that prevented the diseases such as scurvy, beriberi, and pellagra.[1]

Vitamins are calorie-free molecules needed by the body in very small quantities to help with metabolic processes. They are essential, which means they must come from outside the body and be supplied in the food we eat or as a dietary supplement. A common misconception is that "vitamins give you energy." The truth is, vitamins *help* with the metabolic reaction that releases energy within the food molecules, making them the directors of cell processes. But if the body has an adequate supply of vitamins to help with the creation of energy, taking more will not make you more energetic.

Vitamin discovery, both accidental and deliberate, was spread out over 40 years. By 1940, all 13 currently recognized vitamins had been discovered and given a sequential letter of the alphabet. With the discovery and medicinal use of vitamins, thousands of people were cured of debilitating and fatal diseases. Although it is true that vitamins will cure diseases, the specific deficiency must first be present for the vitamin to work its magic. Food for Thought 5-1 itemizes properties of vitamins.

🍎 FOOD FOR THOUGHT 5-1

WHAT ARE VITAMINS?
- Molecules
- Essential
- Organic
- Noncaloric
- Needed in small amounts for cellular metabolism

CATEGORIES OF VITAMINS

Vitamins have alphabet/numeric and common names. Table 5-1 identifies both.

Vitamins are also divided into one of two solvent categories: **water soluble** or **fat soluble**. Water-soluble vitamins include vitamin C and all the B vitamins. Fat-soluble vitamins are A, D, E, and K. Figure 5-1 identifies water-soluble and fat-soluble vitamins.

TABLE 5-1	Properties of Vitamins
Vitamin	**Name**
A	Retinol
B_1	Thiamin
B_2	Riboflavin
B_3	Niacin
B_6	Pyroxidine
B_9	Folate
B_{12}	Cobalamine
H	Biotin
C	Ascorbic acid
D	Calciferol
E	Tocopherol
K	Koagulations

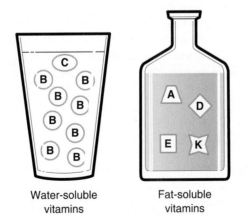

Water-soluble
vitamins

Fat-soluble
vitamins

FIGURE 5-1 Fat-soluble and water-soluble vitamins.

Whether the vitamin is fat soluble or water soluble depends on the following:

- Which foods supply the vitamin
- Vulnerability of the vitamin during cooking
- How the vitamin functions in the body
- Whether the body can store the vitamin

RECOMMENDED NUTRIENT INTAKE

Only minute amounts of any one vitamin are required on a daily basis. Vitamin C has the highest daily requirement of approximately 60 mg. To give you an idea of how much this is: one teaspoon is equivalent to 5,000 mg. It would take 2.5 months worth of the RDI of vitamin C to give you one teaspoonful. Vitamins are found in all food groups, with fruits and vegetables being especially rich. Vitamin B_{12} is the only vitamin found exclusively in animal food, whereas all other vitamins can be obtained from both plants and animals. (See individual vitamins for specific recommended intakes and food sources.)

DIGESTION AND ABSORPTION

Vitamins are *released* from food during the digestive process but are not *digested*.

Water-soluble vitamins (vitamin B complex and C) that are utilized by the body for metabolic processes are absorbed through the small intestine. Any excess that is not used right away is excreted by the kidneys in the urine.

Fat-soluble vitamins (vitamins A, D, E, and K) and fatty acids pass through the small intestine and are absorbed by the body and sent to the lymph system and eventually the blood stream. They are circulated through the blood with the help of lipoproteins.

TOXICITY/IMBALANCE

Eating too many fortified foods or taking a megadose of vitamin supplements—more than the RDI—can produce toxic effects. Fat-soluble vitamins are more toxic than water-soluble vitamins because they can be stored and accumulate in adipose tissues. There is less danger of water-soluble vitamins exerting a toxic effect on the body because storage is limited and usually the excess is excreted on a daily basis.

Vitamin D is the most toxic of all vitamins because of its ultimate effect on the human body. Vitamin D enhances the absorption of calcium, and so an excess of vitamin D causes an excess of calcium circulating in the blood, which is detrimental to the heart.

Two water-soluble vitamins can be somewhat toxic: vitamin B_6 and niacin B_3. Both can have detrimental effects if the amount ingested is more than the kidney can handle and excrete. Food for Thought 5-2 lists the most toxic vitamins.

🍎 FOOD FOR THOUGHT 5-2

TOXICITY

Vitamin D is the most toxic of all vitamins.
Vitamin B_6 is the most toxic *water*-soluble vitamin.

An imbalance of vitamins occurs when too much of one vitamin is added to an adequate diet, causing a deficiency of others. The B complex vitamins function as a group, with one no more important than the other. Excess of one of the B vitamins can throw off the biochemical balance, creating a deficiency in its cofactors. Figure 5-2 illustrates how vitamins function as coenzymes.

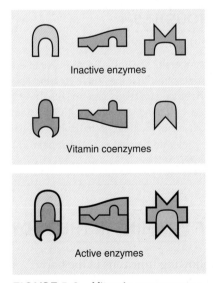

Inactive enzymes

Vitamin coenzymes

Active enzymes

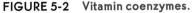

FIGURE 5-2   Vitamin coenzymes.

SYNTHESIZING VITAMINS

If a diet is *in*sufficient in certain vitamins needed for metabolic processes, the body has the capability to manufacture some, but not all. This is accomplished by the body using existing chemicals to **synthesize** vitamins that resemble those we consume in food or supplements. The chemical the body draws on is called a **precursor**. Examples of synthesizing vitamins from precursors are using tryptophan to make niacin (B_3), using a cholesterol compound in skin and sun to make vitamin D, and using carotene to make vitamin A. Once the diet remedies the vitamin deficiency, the body will stop producing the vitamin and use what is supplied in the food. The body can also synthesize vitamin K, biotin, and pantothenic acid with the help of resident bacteria in the colon.

🍎 FOOD FOR THOUGHT 5-3

HOW THE BODY USES PRECURSORS TO MAKE VITAMINS

It uses	To make
Tryptophan	Niacin (B_3)
Cholesterol compound in skin + sun	Vitamin D
Carotene	Vitamin A

🍎 FOOD FOR THOUGHT 5-4

VITAMIN Q

Recently a team of researchers at the Institute of Physical and Chemical Research in Tokyo published a report claiming that they have isolated (pyrroloquinoline quinone) PQQ, with chemical properties similar to vitamin B_6. They believe this discovery is the first new vitamin since 1948 and will include it with vitamins B_2 and B_3, calling it vitamin Q. Currently, PQQ is not included in multivitamin/mineral supplements, but it can be consumed in the diet with parsley, green peppers, kiwi fruit, papaya, spinach, tofu, tea, and certain meats.

PRIMARY ROLE OF VITAMINS IN THE BODY

Vitamins perform the following functions in the body:

- Energy metabolism: B_1 (thiamin), B_2 (riboflavin), B_3 (niacin), biotin, and pantothenic acid help convert calories released from carbohydrates, lipids, and proteins into energy by producing adenosine triphosphate (ATP). ATP is to the body what gas is to a car.

- Tissue synthesis: vitamins A, D, B_6 (pyroxidine), and C help form body cells—epithelium, bone, and collagen.
- Red blood cell (RBC) synthesis: vitamins B_9 (folic acid), B_{12} (cobalamin), E, and K help bone marrow form new RBCs. The life of an RBC is approximately 4 months, so maintenance of an adequate supply demands continual use of body resources. A lack of one or more vitamins at the time of development will manifest as anemia. The type of anemia depends on which vitamin the body is deficient in.
- **Antioxidants**: vitamins A, C, and E serve as protectors from damaging free radicals—oxygen atoms in search of other atoms to attract. As a rule, oxygen travels through the body in pairs. When they disengage and become single, they search for other atoms with which to bond. Once an oxygen atom becomes a free radical, a chain reaction occurs, releasing other oxygen atoms to become free radicals, and body cells get damaged in the process. This cell damage has been blamed for causing certain cancers, arteriosclerosis, cataracts, and other aging diseases because of damage to DNA. Vitamins protect the body by making themselves available to intercept the single oxygen atoms before the chain reaction is set off.

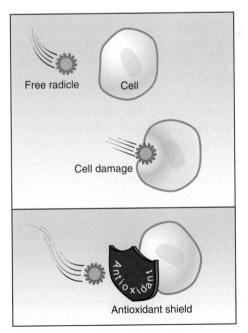

Free radicle   Cell

Cell damage

Antioxidant shield

FIGURE 5-3   Antioxidant action.

TABLE 5-2 Functions of Vitamins	
Function	**Vitamin**
Energy metabolism	Thiamin B_1
	Riboflavin B_2
	Niacin B_3
	Biotin
	Pantothenic acid
Tissue synthesis	A
	D
	Pyroxidine B_6
	C
RBC synthesis	Folate B_9
	B_{12} cyanocobalamine
	E
	K
Antioxidants	A
	C
	E

Vitamin A in its precursor form, beta carotene, is the preferred chemical for antioxidant function. It is the orange-yellow pigment enclosed in fibrous cell walls of plants.

Research for antioxidants is ongoing, so it is important to review the literature frequently to give accurate advice to patients. Presently, there is more support *not* to recommend antioxidants because they may not have the desired effect and can be harmful for some people when taken in large doses.[2–4] Figure 5-3 illustrates how antioxidants protect cells.

Other functions of vitamins include boosting the immune system, keeping the mind alert, helping with hormone production, and synthesizing genetic material. Table 5-2 lists vitamins and their specific functions.

VITAMINS AND FOOD PROCESSING

To ensure that food remains vitamin rich after processing, manufacturers may enrich or fortify their products. **Fortification** occurs when vitamins and minerals are added to the food product, such as in cereals and milk with added vitamins A and D. **Enriched** food products add nutrients that were lost during processing to the level present in the unprocessed product, such as flour, rice, and bread.

Food processing submits ingredients to high temperatures, light, and oxygen—all detrimental to water-soluble vitamins. Boiling food on the stovetop causes nutrients to be released from the food into water; to retain these nutrients, this water can be used to cook something else—for example, rice, mashed potatoes, or soup. Prolonged exposure to heat, as in crockpot cooking, roasting, and frying, can actually destroy water-soluble vitamins. Careful consideration of food preparation can preserve vitamins so that they can benefit the body when consumed in the food. Stir frying at a high temperature seals in nutrients, and short cooking time reduces nutrient loss. Microwaving uses a small amount of water and high temperature for a short amount of time, also preserving most of the vitamins' properties.

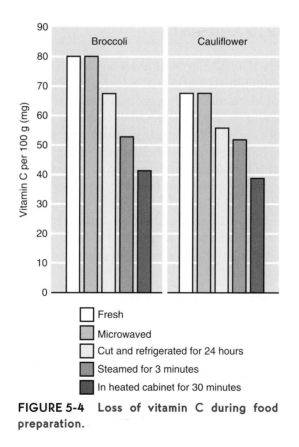

FIGURE 5-4   Loss of vitamin C during food preparation.

The following are some healthful tips when choosing produce to ensure the maximum benefit from the vitamins provided:

- When selecting fresh foods remember that the shorter the time from vine to table, the more nutrients. Nutrient value diminishes as produce ages.
- Shop at roadside stands for homegrown produce that has not been sprayed with chemicals to delay ripening.
- If purchasing produce from the frozen food section in a grocery store, shake the bag to be sure it is not a frozen block of ice. One solid piece in the bag indicates that the product has thawed, which will cause nutrients to leach into the water.
- Canned produce is the least desirable because of intense heat used to sterilize it and the added salt and sugar used to preserve it.

Figure 5-4 illustrates the loss of vitamin C during food preparation.

VITAMIN CHARTS AND LISTS

Most vitamins serve the body in more than one capacity and can be found in multiple foods. Reading charts and lists from textbooks and websites can cause the reader quite a bit of confusion. One source may list a particular vitamin as being involved in blood cell synthesis whereas another might state that the vitamin is needed for 100 different enzyme actions in protein synthesis. Another may list some foods that contain the vitamin whereas yet another may list four new ones. It is almost impossible to make a complete and comprehensive vitamin document, so most references glean important facts and try to arrange them in an organized way. For the purpose of this textbook, an attempt has been made to highlight *major* functions, sources, deficiency and excess states, and RDI. The list is neither comprehensive nor all encompassing, but it can serve as a resource for initial vitamin inquiry. Vitamin information has been organized into water-soluble and fat-soluble categories.

WATER-SOLUBLE VITAMINS

Thiamin: B$_1$

Function

Thiamin functions as a coenzyme in energy metabolism by converting calories released from carbohydrates, lipids, and proteins into energy.

Source

Best source is pork but it is also abundant in fortified cereals and grains, meat, poultry, peanut butter, and eggs.

Deficiency state

Beriberi—symptoms include the following:

- Loss of appetite, muscle weakness, loss of sensation in the extremities, mental confusion
- Enlarged and irregularly beating heart
- Burning tongue, loss of taste
- Occurs in people who eat large amounts of white rice or flour
- Common in alcoholics

Recommended daily intake

Our need for thiamin increases as we consume more carbohydrates and expend more energy. RDI is approximately 1.1 mg.

Riboflavin: B$_2$

Function

Riboflavin helps with production of ATP and releasing energy from carbohydrates, lipids, and proteins.

Source

Sources are milk or milk products (yellow-green fluorescent pigment in milk whey), meat, poultry, fish, and enriched and whole grain breads and cereals.

Deficiency state

Ariboflavinosis—symptoms include the following:

- Tissue inflammation and deterioration
- Angular chelosis: cracks in corners of mouth and lips
- Cracks in skin folds around nose
- Glossitis: atrophy of filiform papillae; swollen, dark red tongue

- Extra blood vessels in cornea with itching, tearing, and sensitivity to light
- Greasy and scaly looking skin

Recommended daily intake

Requirement for riboflavin depends on total calorie intake, energy needs, body size, and growth rate. RDI is around 1.1 mg.

Niacin: B$_3$

Function

Niacin is needed for all cell functions and is a coenzyme and partner to riboflavin. It also converts glucose released from food to energy and assists with blood cell formation.

Source

Meat is a major food source as well as poultry, fish, dark green leafy vegetables, enriched breads and grains, peanuts, beans, and peas.

Deficiency state

Pellagra—symptoms include the following:

- The three Ds: dermatitis (skin turns black when exposed to the sun), diarrhea, and dementia
- Also a fourth D: eventual death

Excess state

- Causes facial flushing
- Decreased blood lipids (popular treatment for high cholesterol in the 1980s)
- Can cause liver damage; chronic overdosing can require a liver transplantation

Recommended daily intake

Recommended intake is approximately 14 mg/day.

Pyroxidine: B$_6$

Function

Pyroxidine functions as a coenzyme in reactions for amino acid, fatty acid, and carbohydrate metabolism. It also assists with formation of blood cells. Pyroxidine gained popularity in the 1980s as a cure for premenstrual syndrome (PMS) and carpal tunnel syndrome but is no longer considered helpful to these syndromes.

Source

Best food sources include anything of animal origin—meat, poultry, fish, pork, liver, and eggs—as well as brown rice, whole wheat, lentils, and peanuts.

Deficiency state

Deficiency states are microcytic anemia, depression, convulsions, depressed immune system, angular chelosis, and glossitis.

Excess state

Vitamin B$_6$ is the most toxic water-soluble vitamin because it can be stored in the muscle and liver. Long-term megadosing may cause permanent neurologic damage that includes numbness in extremities and uncoordinated muscle movement.

Recommended daily intake

The more protein consumed, the more vitamin B$_6$ the body requires. Its bioavailability is affected by 40 different medications, including isoniazid (treatment for tuberculosis). Recommended intake has been set around 1.4 mg/day.

Folate: B$_9$ (Folacin, Folic Acid)

Function

Folate synthesizes amino acids, assists with RBC maturation, and synthesizes DNA and RNA.

Source

Food sources include fortified breads and grains, yeast, kidney, and dark green leafy vegetables. Folate was originally extracted from spinach (folium = leaf).

Deficiency state

Deficiency of B_9 causes fetal neural tube defects and macrocytic anemia. Deficiencies are often seen in alcoholics and found to cause abnormal gastrointestinal (GI) function—irritability, exhaustion, and loss of appetite.

Recommended daily intake

Medications can interfere with bioavailability: aspirin, oral contraceptives, anti-convulsants, and some anticancer drugs. Recommended intake is approximately 400 μg daily.

Cobalamine: B_{12}

Function

Cobalamine converts folate into the form in which it can be used to produce RBCs and nucleic acids for DNA synthesis.

Source

Sources are from animal foods only: meat, poultry, fish, eggs, and dairy products.

Deficiency state

Deficiency in B_{12} may cause pernicious anemia, also known as "macrocytic anemia"; this takes about 5 years to manifest. This is rare but can be found in vegans who eat no animal products. It causes permanent brain and nerve damage, resulting in eventual paralysis of extremities.

Excess state

There are no known toxic side effects from excess ingestion, but because of its pretty red color, it is used in research studies as a placebo.

Recommended daily intake

Recommended intake is approximately 2.4 µg daily.

Biotin: H

Function

Biotin assists in releasing energy from carbohydrates, lipids, and proteins. It also acts as a coenzyme in the synthesis of RNA and DNA.

Source

Bacteria in intestines assist the body in making biotin. Food sources are liver, yeast, legumes, nuts, and egg yolks.

Deficiency state

Deficiency is rare but causes depression, anorexia, nausea, dark red swollen tongue, scaly skin, and hair loss. It has been *mistakenly* presumed by some that if a deficiency causes hair loss, then an excess would cause hair growth. Deficiency is common in geriatric population because of diminished enzymes and acid in the GI tract which inhibits absorption by the body. (See Digestion in Chapter 1.)

Recommended daily intake

This vitamin contains sulfur and is needed in tiny amounts, approximately 30 µg daily.

Pantothenic Acid

Function

Pantothenic acid serves as a coenzyme that assists with the release of energy from carbohydrates, fats, and proteins. It also assists with vitamin D synthesis. It plays a role in melanin production, which protects skin from sun damage.

Source

Pantothenic acid is found everywhere (including the sun) and is in almost every food. It can be manufactured in the intestines by bacteria.

Deficiency state

Because this vitamin is in every living thing, deficiencies are rare. If one does exist, symptoms could include burning feet, fatigue, nausea, poor muscle coordination, and cramping.

Recommended daily intake

Recommended intake has been set at approximately 5 mg daily.

Vitamin C: Ascorbic Acid

Function

Vitamin C assists with collagen formation, strengthens immune system, aids with iron and calcium absorption, and helps with amino acid metabolism. Vitamin C is a natural antihistamine and can shrink swollen tissues. If sinuses are inflamed during a cold or flu, increasing ingestion of vitamin C offers temporary relief from swollen tissues, which gives it its curative reputation.

Source

Food sources are kiwi, citrus fruits, cantaloupe, strawberries, leafy green vegetables, and cruciferous vegetables.

Deficiency state

Scurvy—symptoms include the following:

- Anemia, bleeding gums, nosebleeds, poor digestion, easy bruising
- Merchant seafaring vessels packed limes for daily consumption, giving sailors the nickname of "limeys"

Excess state

The eyes, adrenal glands, and brain have the ability to store high concentrations of vitamin C for about 3 months. Because it can be stored, excesses are possible. Symptoms include the following:

- GI upset
- Diarrhea
- Orange-colored urine

- Interference with anticoagulants
- Iron toxicity

Recommended daily intake

Smokers need to consume two times the amount to compensate the loss from alterations in metabolism. Recommended intake is approximately 60 mg daily.

FAT-SOLUBLE VITAMINS

Vitamin A

Function

Vitamin A assists with formation of epithelium, skin, and mucous membranes. It also maintains healthy eyes and assists with bone remodeling (dismantles existing bone).

Source

Food sources are carrots, yellow and orange fruits and vegetables, spinach and broccoli, liver, eggs, butter, and fortified foods.

Deficiency state

Hypovitaminosis A—symptoms include the following:

- Dry, bumpy skin, poor immunity, slow growth
- Night blindness, xeropthalmia (total blindness)
- Dry epithelium
- Increased incidence of skin, lung, and bladder cancer

Excess state

- Common because of supplements and fortified foods
- Symptoms are headache, vomiting, double vision, hair loss, bone abnormalities, and liver damage

Recommended daily intake

Recommended intake is approximately 800 μg/day.

Vitamin D

Function

Vitamin D is really a hormone that facilitates the absorption of calcium and phosphorus and regulates their presence in plasma. It assists with bone formation by aiding the absorption of calcium.

Source

The body has the ability to manufacture vitamin D from the sun with the use of a cholesterol compound in the skin (fair skinned, 30 minutes; dark skinned, 3 hours). Food sources are fortified milk, liver, egg yolks, and fish oil.

Deficiency state

Rickets (children) and osteomalacia (adult form of rickets); symptoms of rickets include the following:

- Pigeon breasted (prominent sternum) and bow legged (poorly formed bones)
- Nocturnal elevated body temperature (fever)
- Diffuse body soreness and tenderness
- Slight pallor
- Diarrhea
- Liver and spleen enlargement
- Delayed dentition and poorly calcified teeth

Fortified milk eliminated this problem in the United States, but it is still common worldwide. It is most prevalent in extreme climates that keep people inside or keep them wearing clothing that protects them from the sun.

Excess state

The more vitamin D in the body, the more calcium is absorbed and circulating in the bloodstream. Excess calcium collects in soft tissues and can produce calcium stones in the kidneys. It also causes calcifications or hardening of blood vessels, which can be pathologic to the heart.

Symptoms of excess are as follows:

- Nausea, vomiting, and headaches
- Irreversible damage to kidneys and cardiovascular tissue

Recommended daily intake

Recommended intake is approximately 5 to 10 μg daily.

Vitamin E

Function

Vitamin E acts as an antioxidant and protects RBCs.

Source

Sources are margarine and vegetable shortening, salad dressing, whole grains, nuts, and legumes.

Deficiency state

Deficiency is not common but can manifest as hemolytic anemia that causes breakage of RBCs.

Excess state

Vitamin E excess symptoms include the following:

- Nausea
- Diarrhea
- Cramps and bleeding
- Interference with anticoagulant drugs

Recommended daily intake

Recommended intake is approximately 15 mg daily.

Vitamin K

Function

Vitamin K functions as a cofactor for the synthesis of prothrombin required for blood clotting.

Source

It is manufactured by intestinal bacteria; food sources include dark green leafy vegetables.

Deficiency state

Deficiency is caused by diseases that reduce fat absorption or by using broad-spectrum medications that kill intestinal bacteria. Symptoms include prolonged bleeding and increased clotting time, which could result in hemorrhaging.

Excess state

High doses of vitamin K can interfere with anticoagulants.

Recommended daily intake

Recommended intake is approximately 100 µg/day.

Table 5-3 lists the vitamins and their deficiency states.

As a dental health care provider, it is important to know the oral considerations of vitamin deficiencies. Table 5-4 outlines oral deficiency symptoms.

TABLE 5-3	Deficiency States of Vitamins
Vitamin	**Deficiency**
A	Xeropthalmia—night blindness, dry eyes
B_1	Beriberi
B_2	Ariboflavinosis
B_3	Pellagra
B_6	Microcytic anemia—small RBC
B_9	Neural tube defects of fetus
B_{12}	Pernicious anemia
C	Scurvy
D	Rickets—children; osteomalacia—adults
E	Hemolytic anemia—RBC breakage
K	Hemorrhage—failure of blood to clot

TABLE 5-4	Oral Deficiency Symptoms
Vitamin	Oral Deficiency Symptoms
A	Xerostomia Oral leukoplakia Hyperkeratosis Hyperplastic gingival tissue
B	Red swollen lips with vertical fissures and chelosis Burning, smooth, red tongue, which may be ulcerated, geographic, with atrophied papillae Red, ulcerated, burning gingival tissues
C	Red-purplish, swollen, bleeding gums Loose teeth Slow healing
D	Failure of bone wounds to heal Enamel hypocalcification Loss of alveolar bone Thinning of trabeculation
E	No known deficiency symptoms
K	Failure of wounds to stop bleeding

COUNSELING PATIENTS

The following tips are taken from the Mayo Clinic website and may be of interest to your patients when discussing vitamins:

- "Supplements are not substitutes." There is no substitute for wholesome foods that supply other nutrients like complex carbohydrates, fiber, and other phytochemicals.
- Synthetic supplements are the same as "natural" vitamins, so there is no need to pay a lot for supplements. The body does not recognize the difference between natural and synthetic vitamins.
- Never take more than 100% of the RDI of any one vitamin. Megadosing on supplements increases your body's need for that nutrient, and cutting back

to the required level may cause a pseudodeficiency. When you increase intake of one vitamin, you need to increase its cofactors.

• Store vitamin supplements in a cool, dry place. Never place or store the container in a hot or humid place such as the bathroom.

If the patient has a health problem, always check with a doctor, pharmacist, or registered dietitian first. Some vitamins react negatively with medical conditions. For example, high doses of niacin can harm the liver, vitamins E and K interfere with anticoagulants, men who drink alcohol and take beta carotene have a higher incidence of prostate cancer, and smokers who take beta carotene have an increased incidence of lung cancer.

Putting This Into Practice

1. Vitamins should dissolve in the stomach within 30 minutes to make them available to the body when they pass to the small intestines. If they do not dissolve with help from hydrochloric acid in the stomach within this time, they can pass through to the intestines whole and will not be available for use by the body. Find out if your vitamin supplement will pass this test; cover your vitamin supplement with vinegar and check back in 30 minutes.
2. Compare an inexpensive brand of vitamins to a more expensive brand for vitamin content. Place the labels side by side and determine if the bottles contain the same number and percentage of vitamins.

WEB RESOURCES

Center for Disease Control and Prevention—Folic Acid Now, Before You Know You're Pregnant http://www.cdc.gov/ncbddd/fact/folnow.htm

Dispelling Fears of Vitamin D Toxicity http://www.cholecalciferol-council.com/toxicity.pdf

Mayo Clinic—Drugs and Supplements Information
http://www.mayoclinic.com/findinformation/druginformation/listinvoke.cfm?range=U-Wz

MedlinePlus Medical Encyclopedia—Vitamins
http://www.nlm.nih.gov/medlineplus/ency/article/002399.htm

National Institute of Health—Facts About B6

http://www.cc.nih.gov/ccc/supplements/vitb6.html

National Institute of Health—Facts About Folate

http://www.cc.nih.gov/ccc/supplements/folate.html

U.S. Food and Drug Administration—Folic Acid Fortification

http://vm.cfsan.fda.gov/~dms/wh-folic.html

REFERENCES

1. Funk C. *The Vitamins*. Baltimore, MD: Williams and Wilkins; 1922.
2. Hasnain BI, Mooradian AD. Recent trials of antioxidant therapy: what should we be telling our patients?. *Cleve Clin J Med* 2004;71(4):327–334.
3. Hlubik P, Sstritecka H. Antioxidants–clinical aspects. *Cent Eur J Public Health* 2004;12: S28–S30.
4. Stanner SA, Hughes J, Kelly CNM, et al. A review of the epidemiological evidence for the "antioxidant hypothesis". *Public Health Nutr* 2004;7(3):407–422.

SUGGESTED READING

Abraham J, Smith HL, eds. *Regulation of the Pharmaceutical Industry*. London: Palgrave; 2003.

Asimov I. *The Chemicals of Life*. New York: Abelard-Schuman; 1954.

Combs G. *The Vitamins*. San Diego, CA: Academic Press; 1992.

Is your supplement dissolving? *Tufts University Health NutrLett* 1977;15(9).

Liebman B. Do you know your vitamin ABC's? *Nutr Action Health Lett* 1999;26(7).

Liebman B. Antioxidants. *Nutr Action Health Lett* 2002.

Shills M, ed. *Modern Nutrition in Health and Disease*, 10th ed. Lippincott Williams & Wilkins; 2006.

Smith R, Olson R, eds. *The Biographical Encyclopedia of Scientists*. New York: Marshall Cavendish Corporation; 1998.

Touger-Decker R. *Oral manifestations of nutrient deficiencies* 1998;65(5/6):355–361.

Vitamins and minerals: how much is too much? *Nutr Action Health Lett* 2001;28(5).

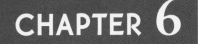

CHAPTER 6

MINERALS

OBJECTIVES

Upon completion of the chapter, the reader will be able to:

1 List seven major minerals
2 Define the difference between a major and trace mineral
3 State five functions of minerals in the body
4 Discuss the function of a sodium pump and name the minerals involved in the process
5 Outline the cycle of minerals in the ecosystem
6 Outline the digestive process of minerals
7 Using a chart, identify mineral excess and deficiency as well as roles, recommended daily intake (RDI), and sources

KEY TERMS

Anions
Bioavailability
Cations
Extracellular
Goiter

Heme Iron
Hemochromatosis
Homeostasis
Intracellular
Ionic Compound

Major Mineral
Methylmercury
Nonheme Iron
Osmosis
Trace Mineral

Major Minerals AT A GLANCE*

Major Minerals	Major Functions	RDI/Day (Adult)	Food Source	Deficiency State	Excess States
Calcium	Mineralization of calcified structures Contracting muscles Nerve conduction Cofactor in blood-clotting protein	1,200 mg	Dairy Animal bones Stone-ground meal Tofu Broccoli Legumes Fortified orange juice	Rickets Osteomalacia Osteoporosis	
Chloride	Anion that partners with sodium to maintain extracellular water balance	750 mg	Table salt Processed foods Meat Eggs	Rare	
Magnesium	Mineralization of calcified structures Protein synthesis Neuromuscular activity	400 mg	Nuts Meat Green leafy vegetables Legumes Grains	Occurs from dieting, gastric bypass, drinking soft water, or loss during body functions; causes muscle spasms, hallucinations, mental derangement	Occurs with long-term antacid use
Phosphorous	Mineralization of calcified structures Energy metabolism Protein synthesis Muscle contractions	700 mg	Meat Eggs Fish Poultry Legumes Dairy	Occurs with use of antacids	

*Major Minerals** AT A GLANCE (continued)

Major Minerals	Major Functions	RDI/Day (Adult)	Food Source	Deficiency State	Excess States
Potassium	Cation that works to balance fluid inside cells Muscle contractions Neurologic transmissions	2,000 mg	Processed food Meat Grains Fruits and vegetables	Occurs during dehydration Muscle cramps Cardiac arrest Respiratory failure	Numbness of extremities, face, and tongue Dilation of heart
Sodium	Cation in extracellular fluid for regulation of fluid balance	500 mg	Table salt Processed foods Meat Eggs Dairy	Rare	Hypertension
Sulfur	Part of biotin and thiamin Part of enzymes that detoxify Liver function Acid–base balance of body fluid	None	Meat Poultry Fish Legumes	Rare	Rare

NIH, National Institutes of Health; RDI, recommended daily intake.
* (Based on National Institutes of Health Medline Plus)

Usually when one discusses vitamins, the mention of minerals is not far behind. Since they are combined in daily dietary supplements, it seems that they are inseparable. Minerals, like vitamins, are essential chemical elements. They are different, however, in that they are metals with electrical charges, not separate molecules; are inorganic (whereas vitamins are organic); and are noncaloric because they do not contain carbon. Many necessary minerals are provided in food and water and are found within our body's water content. We need to replace minerals every day by eating food or drinking water, making use of the minerals we need and excreting those that we do not need. The body must be efficient in balancing minerals because excess of one can cause an imbalance of another, leading to disease. Food for Thought 6-1 identifies factors of minerals.

🍎 **FOOD FOR THOUGHT 6-1**

WHAT ARE MINERALS?

- Essential
- Inorganic
- Noncaloric
- Metals
- Small electrically charged particles

CATEGORIES OF MINERALS

There are two categories of minerals: major and trace, depending on body needs. Major minerals are needed in quantities greater than 100 mg/day and trace minerals are needed in quantities less than 100 mg/day. Following are the seven major minerals:

1. Calcium
2. Chloride
3. Magnesium
4. Phosphorus
5. Potassium
6. Sodium
7. Sulfur

More than 30 trace minerals have been identified as essential to life. Some of the more common trace minerals are as follows:

1. Chromium
2. Cobalt
3. Copper
4. Fluoride
5. Iodine
6. Iron
7. Lithium
8. Manganese
9. Molybdenum
10. Nickel
11. Selenium
12. Silicone
13. Tin
14. Vanadium
15. Zinc

PRIMARY ROLE OF MINERALS IN THE BODY

As with vitamins, the body needs minerals for many metabolic functions. Making up 4% of the body's mass, minerals are found in hormones and enzymes and assist the body in the following ways:

- Controlling water balance, muscle contraction, and nerve transmission: Sodium, potassium, and chloride control fluid inside and outside our body cells and maintain exchange of nutrients and waste. Fluid compartments are either intracellular (within a cell) or extracellular (outside the cell wall). Metabolic work takes place inside the cells, and fluid outside the cells transports nutrients and waste throughout the body. Water is constantly passing in and out of cell membranes with the help of electrically charged minerals such as sodium, potassium, and chloride. This is sometimes referred to as the "pumping action" that maintains homeostasis—water balance—within and between our cells.
- Tissue synthesis: Iron, calcium, phosphorous, and magnesium assist with the formation of teeth, bones, and blood. Zinc assists with the synthesis of eye pigment needed for night vision and the formation of collagen tissue.
- Energy metabolism: Phosphorus precipitates energy metabolism and is part of adenosine triphosphate (ATP). It is also part of lipoproteins, which transport lipids in blood.
- Essential cofactors in chemical reactions: Copper and iron work together to aid with the synthesis of hemoglobin.
- Facilitators in the antioxidant process: Selenium and sulfur work in tandem with vitamins A, C, and E, bonding with free oxygen radicals to avoid cell destruction.

MINERALS IN THE ECOSYSTEM

As with vitamins, there is no best food source that contains all minerals. A varied diet with selections from all food groups, specifically unrefined foods, will ensure an adequate intake. All essential minerals are ingested through our diets—through drinking water and our food choices. Minerals are found in oceans, lakes, and rivers as well as in the soil where our food is grown. They enter the food chain by way of plants absorbing them from the soil and water and animals eating the plant. To complete the cycle, decaying plants and animals return minerals to the soil. The minerals end up on our table in the food we eat and the beverages we drink. Figure 6-1 illustrates the mineral cycle.

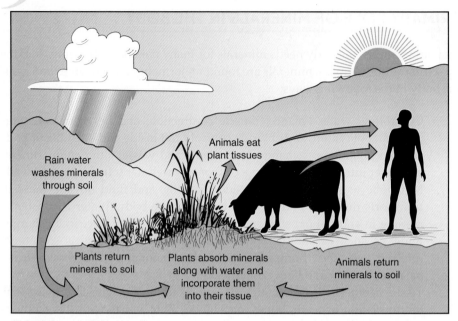

FIGURE 6-1　The mineral cycle.

DIGESTION

Minerals, like vitamins, are not digested but released from foods during the digestive process, making them available for use in the body's many metabolic functions. Once released, they are absorbed by the body through the villi in the small intestine. Minerals not utilized are filtered through the kidneys and excreted in the urine.

BIOAVAILABILITY

Bioavailability means that a mineral is available for the body to use for metabolic functions. Increasing intake of one mineral can affect how others get absorbed as they compete with each other for bioavailability. For example, taking more than the recommended dose of zinc can affect the absorption of copper, and increasing calcium intake may alter the body's absorption of iron. Also, phytochemicals known as "phylates" and "oxylates," found in certain foods, can bind with minerals and make them unavailable to the body. Food for Thought 6-2 identifies minerals affected by these chemicals.

> ## 🍎 FOOD FOR THOUGHT 6-2
>
> ### PHYLATES AND OXYLATES
>
> - Phylates and oxylates bind with minerals and prevent their absorption.
> - Phylates are found in fiber and bind with zinc.
> - Oxylates are found in leafy greens and bind with calcium.

MINERAL IONS

If an electron is added or removed from a neutral atom, it forms an ion. Minerals can be either positively charged cations (+) or negatively charged anions (−). An ionic compound is made of a combination of positive and negative ions. Many dietary minerals appear in the ionic form, switching the "ine" suffix to "ide." Examples are fluorine becoming fluoride and chlorine becoming chloride. Metal anions team up with cations, forming ionic compounds in food. A good example is sodium and chloride making salt. You may see the minerals named in textbooks as either the element or ion, but for the purpose of this text, they will be referred to as the "ion."

MINERAL DEFICIENCY

A carefully chosen diet will provide an abundance of all minerals needed for daily metabolism, making supplements unnecessary. Occasionally, deficiencies do exist because of diets that restrict or eliminate foods rich in the following minerals: calcium, potassium, iron, zinc, and magnesium. Those who are lactose intolerant (see Chapter 2) may eliminate calcium-rich dairy products from their diets, creating a deficiency in calcium. People with anorexia nervosa, who are on severe calorie-restricted diets, eventually develop a deficiency in potassium. Because of monthly blood loss, many young women are found to be deficient in iron. Strict vegetarians (vegans) who eliminate all forms of animal products and who are not efficient in combining proteins may develop a deficiency in zinc. Severe alcoholics who choose drinking alcohol over eating will develop a deficiency in magnesium over time. A deficiency in each of these minerals will manifest their own set of symptoms. (See specific minerals for a list of deficiency symptoms.) Food for Thought 6-3 lists common mineral deficiencies.

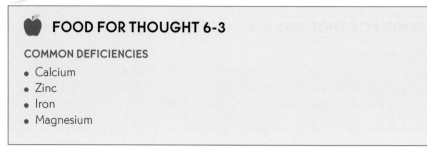

MINERAL EXCESS

Processed foods are the bane of our existence. The convenience of packaged, canned, and microwavable food makes them a daily staple, but consumers should beware: Processed foods have an abundance of sodium and chloride. Sodium and chloride together make table salt, which is used as a preservative; salt draws fluid out of bacteria, rendering it ineffective. These two minerals are blamed for an increased incidence in hypertension for those who are salt sensitive. Ingesting an excess of many minerals can have a toxic effect on the body, although potentially toxic minerals are less absorbable than those with a low potential for toxicity.

MINERALS THAT FUNCTION AS ELECTROLYTES

Osmosis is when fluid passes freely from one side of a permeable membrane to another. The "sodium pump" in the human body works by osmosis, with fluid being equalized on both sides by electrical charges inside and outside cells. Sodium (+) and chloride (−) work together outside the cell wall and potassium (+) works within. Food for Thought 6-4 lists minerals that are considered electrolytes.

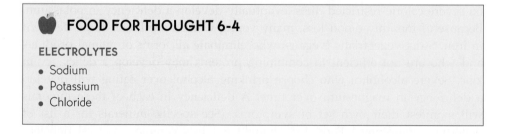

Sodium (Na⁺)

Function

Sodium is a soft silvery metal and is one of the two elements of table salt. It is used liberally as a food additive for flavoring, as a preservative, and to flavor baking soda. It functions as a cation (positive charge) in extracellular fluid to regulate fluid balance.

Sources

Sources include table salt, meat, eggs, dairy products, unprocessed produce and grains, legumes, and most processed foods.

Recommended daily intake

The RDI would fit in the palm of your hand. The suggested daily minimum, 500 mg, includes sodium added during processing and after preparation; most diets, however, average around 2,000 mg. An intake of a quarter teaspoon per day is safe, with an upper intake of no more than one and a quarter teaspoon per day.

Figure 6-2 illustrates recommended sodium intake.

Deficiency and excess

Because of its widespread use in processed food, deficiency is rare and excess more common. Disease of excess is hypertension.

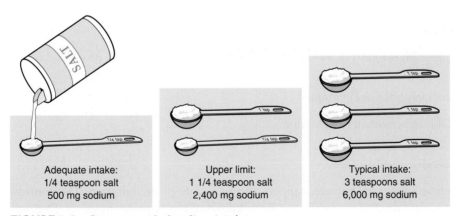

Adequate intake:	Upper limit:	Typical intake:
1/4 teaspoon salt	1 1/4 teaspoon salt	3 teaspoons salt
500 mg sodium	2,400 mg sodium	6,000 mg sodium

FIGURE 6-2   **Recommended sodium intake.**

Chloride (Cl⁻)

Function

Chloride is the partner to sodium in table salt. Together they work in extracellular fluid to maintain the body's fluid balance.

Source

Sources include table salt, meat, fish, eggs, and processed foods.

Recommended daily intake

Recommended daily consumption is approximately 750 mg.

Deficiency

Deficiency is rare because of its abundance in processed foods.

Potassium (K⁺)

Function

Potassium is the "man on the inside" found in intracellular fluid, working with sodium and chloride on the "outside" in extracellular fluid to maintain water balance in the body's fluid compartments. It plays an essential role in muscle contractions and neurologic transmissions

Source

Potassium is found in meats, grains, fruits and vegetables, and processed foods.

Recommended daily intake

RDI is approximately 2,000 mg.

Deficiency and excess

Deficiency is rare but can happen during a state of dehydration. The confusion from dehydration prevents one from knowing that a problem exists. Deficiency symptoms are also apparent in those whose diets are severely restricted. Symptoms of deficiency include the following:

- Nausea and vomiting
- Listlessness
- Muscle cramps
- Cardiac arrest
- Respiratory failure

Excess can cause the following symptoms:

- Numbness of extremities, face, and tongue
- Muscle weakness
- Cardiac arrhythmias: the heart will dilate and quit contracting

Food for Thought 6-5 explains the importance of adequate potassium when taking diuretic medication.

🍎 FOOD FOR THOUGHT 6-5

DIURETICS

Potassium is lost in the urine when a person is placed on diuretics to help lower blood pressure. Diuretics rid the body of fluid so that less pressure is placed on the vessels, thereby reducing blood pressure. Many patients who are on diuretics are instructed by their physician to eat a banana or drink a glass of orange juice every day to replenish lost potassium.

MINERALS FOR ENERGY METABOLISM

Food for Thought 6-6 lists minerals needed for energy metabolism.

🍎 FOOD FOR THOUGHT 6-6

MINERALS FOR ENERGY METABOLISM

- Phosphorus
- Magnesium
- Manganese
- Iodine
- Chromium

Phosphorus (P)

Function

Phosphorus assists with the formation of teeth and bones: Eighty percent of the phosphorus in the body is stored in teeth and bones. It also acts as an enzyme in energy metabolism and protein synthesis and is necessary for muscle contractions.

Source

Food sources are anything that is protein-rich: meat, eggs, poultry, fish, legumes, and dairy products.

Recommended daily intake

RDI is around 700 mg.

Deficiency and excess

Deficiency can happen if a person consumes antacids: Many antacids contain aluminum, which competes with phosphorus for absorption (bioavailability). If aluminum-containing antacids are consumed over a long period of time, changes in bone density, such as osteoporosis and osteomalacia, may occur.

Magnesium (Mg)

Function

Magnesium is a silver-white metallic mineral essential for mineralization of bones and teeth: Sixty percent is stored in bones and teeth, 39% in soft tissues, and 1% in extracellular fluid. It also assists with protein synthesis and neuromuscular activity and is a cofactor in utilization of ATP.

Source

Food sources are green leafy vegetables, nuts, meats, legumes, and grains.

Recommended daily intake

RDI is approximately 400 mg.

Deficiency and excess

Dieting and gastric bypass surgery can affect the absorption of magnesium, as can drinking "soft" water devoid of the mineral. The body can "sweat out" magnesium during excess exercise and lose it during bouts of chronic diarrhea and alcoholism.[1] Symptoms of magnesium deficiency include nausea, muscle spasms, hallucinations, and mental derangement. High calcium intake can depress absorption of magnesium (bioavailability competition). Excess can occur from long-term use of antacids listing magnesium as an ingredient.

Manganese (Mn)

Function

Manganese is needed for many enzyme reactions. It also helps metabolize carbohydrates and assists in synthesizing bones of inner ear.

Source

Food sources are plants and grains.

Recommended daily intake

RDI is approximately 2 mg.

Deficiency and excess

Deficiency in manganese is associated with poor reproduction rates, growth retardation, skeletal abnormalities, and bad balance. Excess has been noted in miners who are environmentally exposed to high levels of manganese and exhibit the following symptoms: Parkinson's disease, speech impairment, headaches, and leg cramps.

Iodide (I)

Function

Iodide is part of the hormone thyroxin that regulates our pace of work and mental development.

Source

Sources of iodide are iodized salt, seawater, and seafood.

Recommended daily intake

RDI is approximately 150 µg.

Deficiency and excess

A deficiency will manifest as a **goiter**, which appears as an enlarged thyroid gland. Symptoms would be those related to decreased thyroid hormone function—hypothyroidism: weight gain, dry skin and hair, low blood pressure, intolerance of cold, and lethargy. Figure 6-3 illustrates a goiter.

Myxedema is another deficiency condition that happens when the thyroid gland decreases its absorption of iodine or there is not enough supplied in the diet. It manifests with decreased metabolic rate, slow and slurred speech, enlarged tongue, swollen hands, brittle hair, drowsiness, and increased sensitivity to cold temperatures.

Chromium (Cr)

Function

Chromium is essential for glucose and energy metabolism. It is a cofactor in insulin production and needed for uptake of insulin by cell membranes.

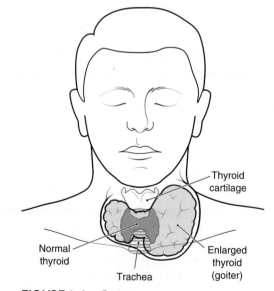

FIGURE 6-3   Goiter.

Source

In the diet, chromium is found in whole grains, beer, fats and oil, meat, yeast, mushrooms, and prunes.

Recommended daily intake

RDI is approximately 30 mg.

Deficiency and excess

Deficiency in chromium may resemble diabetes in that it results in poor glucose tolerance. This is seen more in patients on intravenous feedings.

MINERALS NEEDED FOR TISSUE SYNTHESIS

Food for Thought 6-7 lists minerals that help with tissue synthesis.

🍎 FOOD FOR THOUGHT 6-7

MINERALS NEEDED FOR TISSUE SYNTHESIS

- Calcium
- Fluoride
- Zinc
- Phosphorous
- Magnesium

Calcium (Ca$^+$)

Function

Calcium is the most abundant mineral in the body, with 99% found in teeth and bones. A growing body needs calcium to build healthy teeth and bones. The other 1%, available in blood and soft tissue, is used for conducting nerve signals, contracting muscles, keeping cell membranes permeable, forming bridges between collagen strands, and acting as cofactor in the synthesis of blood-clotting protein. These physiologic needs of calcium are so vital to survival that the body will actually take calcium from bone to support these functions, before it uses it to maintain bones.

Although bones may appear to be hard, static structures, calcium is constantly being removed and replaced. As the body ages, the ability to absorb calcium is diminished. Children can absorb around 75% of the calcium supplied in their diets, whereas adults can absorb only about 25%. In anticipation of this decreased absorption, calcium is stored in bones, creating a "warehouse of calcium," until the age of 35 when absorption and storage ability are reduced. The body has the capability of storing about 10 years' worth of calcium for future bone remodeling and physiologic functions. Figure 6-4 diagrams rate of calcium loss.

Source

Think "Milk—Bones—Stones." Best food sources are dairy products, animal bones such as sardines, stone-ground cornmeal and lime-processed tortillas, tofu, broccoli, and legumes. Orange juice with added calcium is also a very good daily source.

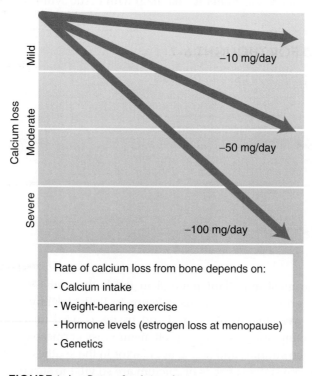

FIGURE 6-4   **Rate of calcium loss.**

Recommended daily intake

A 1,200 mg RDI has been suggested for maintenance of healthy bones and physiologic function.

Deficiency and excess

If calcium is deficient in the diet during the growth years, the result is reduced bone mineralization. Osteomalacia means "soft bones." When this occurs in children it is called "rickets," which is the deficiency disease of vitamin D. Because vitamin D assists the body in absorbing calcium, the two are symbiotic. (See Chapter 5 for vitamin D deficiency state.) Osteoporosis is a disease where there is not enough calcium to maintain bone, resulting in a net loss of structure. The importance of storing calcium in the teenage years should be emphasized to reduce the risk of osteoporosis and bone fractures. The disease proceeds faster in women after menopause because of the decrease in estrogen production.[2,3] Weight-bearing activity puts stress on bones, helping them retain calcium and decreasing resorption. Figures 6-5 and 6-6 illustrate the threshold for bone breakage and osteoporosis, respectively.

It was once believed that calcium supplements increased the incidence of kidney stones. Recent studies have shown that normal calcium intake with supplementation does not contribute to this risk.[4-6]

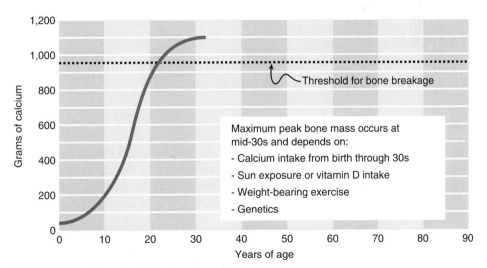

FIGURE 6-5   Threshold for bone breakage.

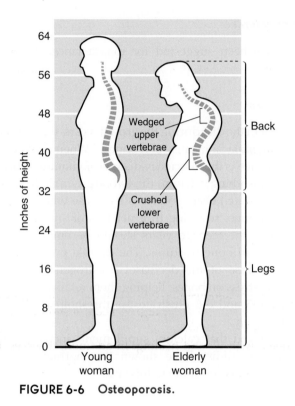

FIGURE 6-6 Osteoporosis.

Fluoride (F)

Fluoride is the only mineral that is considered nonessential. We do not need to include it in our diet for important physiologic functions.

Function

Fluoride increases retention of calcium in teeth and bones. If consumed by the pregnant woman or infant, it becomes incorporated into the developing tooth structure. The hydroxyl ion in the tooth combines with the fluoride ion to form fluorohydroxyapatite, which makes the structure less soluble and more resistant to demineralization.

Source

Fluoride is found in drinking water, soil, tea, and seafood.

Recommended daily intake

Because fluoride is nonessential, there is no RDI; however, a daily intake of approximately 3 mg can prevent defective enamel development.

Deficiency and excess

A fluoride deficiency correlates with increased incidence of dental caries. An excess of fluoride during tooth development can manifest as dental fluorosis: This appears clinically as mottled enamel or enamel hypoplasia, which is incomplete development of tooth enamel because of inadequate calcium and phosphate metabolism.[7]

Zinc (Zn)

Function

Zinc assists in protein metabolism, synthesizing DNA during cell division, and development of pigment needed for night vision; it aids in immune response and with insulin storage in the pancreas. Zinc is also involved in taste and smell sensitivity and helps with wound healing. In addition, it serves as a cofactor in more than 200 enzyme systems.

Source

Meat, poultry, and fish offer more bioavailable zinc than plant sources.

Recommended daily intake

RDI is approximately 10 mg.

Deficiency and excess

A deficiency in zinc can cause anorexia (loss of appetite), slow tissue repair, night blindness, mental lethargy, and a loss of taste and smell. An excess of zinc can interfere with copper absorption, alter cholesterol metabolism, and weaken blood vessels. Toxicity can occur in people who eat food cooked in galvanized pots and pans.

MINERALS NEEDED FOR RED BLOOD CELL SYNTHESIS

Food for Thought 6-8 lists minerals that synthesize red blood cells.

> ### 🍎 FOOD FOR THOUGHT 6-8
>
> **MINERALS NEEDED FOR RED BLOOD CELL SYNTHESIS**
> - Iron
> - Copper

Iron (Fe)

Function

About 20% of the iron in the body is stored in bone marrow, the liver, and the spleen to act as a reserve in times of iron depletion. The rest of the iron in the body can be found in the blood. The iron in hemoglobin binds with oxygen in the lungs and carries it to other cells in the body, where it is exchanged for carbon dioxide.

Source

The source of iron in the diet makes a difference in its bioavailability. More iron is absorbed from animals (40%) than plants (10%). Iron from animal sources is called "heme iron" and from plant sources is called "nonheme."

- Heme iron food sources include meat, fish, and poultry.
- Nonheme iron is found in egg yolks, leafy greens, and legumes.

Vitamin C helps with absorption of iron. Drinking orange juice or including other foods rich in vitamin C can enhance the uptake of iron from the meal.

Recommended daily intake

RDI is 8 mg for men and 18 mg for women.

Deficiency and excess

Iron is usually well conserved in the body because the kidneys will not excrete it. Iron stores can be depleted during bleeding from any cause—including menstruation, bleeding ulcer, or severe wounds. Females can lose up to 45 mg of iron during menstruation. This along with a poor diet accounts for up to 50% of American women exhibiting iron deficiencies. Iron deficiency anemia is one of the most prevalent world nutritional problems.

Anemia is detected through a blood test that shows hemoglobin levels less than needed to supply the oxygen demands of the body. There will be a decrease in the number of red blood cells and low plasma levels. Symptoms of anemia are as follows:

- Pallor
- Angular cheilosis
- Lethargy
- Apathy
- Short attention span
- Irritability

Iron is the most toxic mineral because the body has the capacity to store it. Excess absorption occurs with overconsumption of vitamin C. Hemochromatosis is a hereditary disease where there is increased iron absorption from the small intestines.[8]

Copper (Cu)

Function

Copper aids the absorption of iron and with iron, works to synthesize hemoglobin. Copper is also needed for regulating blood lipid levels and assists with collagen formation and nerve function.

Source

Food sources include liver, whole grains, nuts, legumes, vegetables, fruit, water from copper water pipes, and chocolate cooked in copper pots.

Recommended daily intake

The RDI is approximately 1.5 mg.

Deficiency and excess

Deficiencies are rare but can happen with excess intake of zinc, because these two minerals compete for bioavailability.

ANTIOXIDANTS

Food for Thought 6-9 lists minerals that assist in the antioxidant process.

🍎 FOOD FOR THOUGHT 6-9

ANTIOXIDANTS
- Selenium
- Sulfur

Selenium (Se)

Function

Selenium is a trace mineral that works with vitamin E as an antioxidant.

Source

Food sources depend on the abundance of selenium in soil and animals that eat plants grown in the soil. Because of this it is geographically higher in some areas than others. Foods containing selenium are grains, vegetables, and meats.

Recommended daily intake

RDI is approximately 60 μg.

Deficiency and excess

A selenium deficiency can cause cardiac weakness. An excess can cause hair loss, fatigue, and vomiting.

Sulfur (S)

Function

Sulfur is part of the vitamins biotin and thiamin. It is also found in enzymes that are part of the body's drug-detoxifying pathway. Sulfur is needed for liver function and also to maintain the acid–base balance of body fluid.

Source

Food sources include meat, poultry, fish, and legumes; it is also found in food preservatives.

Recommended daily intake

There is no RDI for sulfur.

Deficiency and excess

There are no known deficiency or toxicity states.

NONNUTRITIVE MINERAL INGESTION

Lead and mercury are two minerals that are highly toxic. Although their addition to one's diet is not intentional, they enter the body inadvertently by ingestion or absorption through the skin.

Lead (Pb)

Lead is a soft blue-gray metallic element that is used to make batteries, solder seals, wheel weights, TV tubes, foil or wire, x-ray shields, soundproofing material, and ammunition. It is very toxic and can be ingested by drinking water that flows through lead-soldered water pipes or by consuming food prepared in lead cookware and lead crystal. It can also be inhaled from household dust and air or pass through the skin from soil or hair dye. Two commercial products, paint and gasoline, included lead in their ingredients but have reconfigured their formulas, thereby reducing the incidence of lead poisoning. The greatest source of lead poisoning is still from deteriorating paint used in residential housing before 1978. Paint formulas prior to this date included lead, which gave the paint a sweet taste and made it desirable for children to eat chipped paint. Until recently, lead in gasoline controlled the "knocking" in engines. Inhaling exhaust fumes or the air around busy highways contributed to many cases of lead poisoning. Effects of lead poisoning include reduced IQ, learning disabilities, stunted growth, impaired hearing, memory and concentration problems, fertility problems, and nerve disorders.

Mercury (Hg)

Mercury, also called "quicksilver," is a shiny metallic liquid that beads up and can be made to roll around. It is not required for any metabolic functions. Mercury is found naturally in the environment and is released into the atmosphere through industrial pollution. Particles fall through the air into bodies of water, where it turns into methylmercury. Fish living in rivers and streams absorb methylmercury, which can then be consumed by humans. Although the human body can tolerate small amounts of mercury, it can be a health concern for certain groups of people. Nervous systems of infants, growing fetuses, and young children with small body mass can be harmed by ingesting too much methylmercury. Fish and shellfish, with their omega-3 fatty acids and high protein content, have many healthful benefits and should not be completely eliminated from the diet. The U.S. Department of Health and Human Services has suggested eating smaller and younger fish to eliminate mercury and choosing more fish from the low-mercury category.

- Fish with high levels of mercury are shark, swordfish, king mackerel, or tilefish.
- Fish low in mercury are shrimp, canned tuna (albacore has more mercury than canned light tuna), salmon, pollock, and catfish.

See Food for Thought 6-10 for an example of how mercury was used in the hat industry.

Mercury is also found in thermometers, medications, laboratory chemicals, and dental amalgam. Increased concern about the effect of mercury on the body revolves around it being released from dental amalgam during placement. This appears to be a worldwide concern, as research continues to discover a relationship between mercury absorption and disease processes. The American Dental Association's position remains that dental amalgam is safe because mercury binds with silver, copper, and tin into a hard, stable substance.

🍎 FOOD FOR THOUGHT 6-10

MAD AS A HATTER

Salt of mercury was once used to flatten felt on hats. Workers in this industry had a higher incidence of a cluster of symptoms: tremors, drooling, and paranoia. This is where the phrase "mad as a hatter" originated.

COUNSELING PATIENTS

Consider the following when counseling patients:

- Use the same caution in purchasing minerals as with vitamins (see Counseling Patients section in Chapter 5).
- Excessive use of processed food may lead to:
  - Deficiencies of calcium, iron, and zinc
  - Excess of sodium and chloride
- When preparing food:
  - Although minerals are not destroyed by heat, boiling and stewing cause leaching into surrounding fluid. Use this fluid to prepare rice, mashed potatoes, pasta, and so on
  - Steaming and stir frying retain minerals.
  - Be frugal when adding salt to a prepared meal.
  - Cast-iron cookware adds absorbable iron, especially when cooking acidic foods like tomatoes.

Putting This Into Practice

1. Place the labels from the box, package, can, or bottle of your favorite processed foods in front of you. Read the list of ingredients and locate as many minerals as you can. Write down all the minerals that are more than half the daily recommended allowance.
2. Check the label of your daily multivitamin/mineral supplement to determine which minerals and their percentage of RDI it contains. Add the percentage of the minerals in the supplement with the percentage contained in your favorite processed foods to determine your daily consumption.
3. Which minerals are you consuming in excess?
4. Which minerals are deficient in your diet?

WEB RESOURCES

Center for Disease Control—Childhood Lead Poisoning Prevention Program
   http://www.cdc.gov/nceh/lead/lead.htm

Food and Drug Administration, Department of Health and Human Services—Health Care
   Claims: Sodium and Hypertension http://vm.cfsan.fda.gov/~lrd/cf101-74.html

GlaxoSmithKline Calcium Information http://www.calciuminfo.com

HealthWorld Online, American Institute of Preventive Medicine—Women's Health:
   Anemia http://www.healthy.net/scr/article.asp?PageType=article&ID=1211

Information From the Heart Foundation—Salt and Hypertension
   http://www.heartfoundation.com.au/downloads/salt_and_hypertension.pdf

The Linus Pauling Institute—Micronutrient Information Center: Calcium
   http://lpi.oregonstate.edu/infocenter/minerals/calcium/

Mercury Poisoning News http://www.mercurypoisoningnews.com/

National Dairy Council—Nutrition and Product Information
   http://www.nationaldairycouncil.org/nutrition/index.asp

National Institute of Health—FactsAbout Zinc
   http://www.cc.nih.gov/ccc/supplements/zinc.html

National Osteoporosis Foundation—Calcium and Vitamin D
   http://www.nof.org/prevention/calcium.htm

National Safety Council—Fact Sheet Library: Lead Poisoning
   http://www.nsc.org/library/facts/lead.htm

Salt Institute—Citizen Petition: Reaction to the FDA's Paper on Sodium and Hypertension
   http://www.saltinstitute.org/pubstat/petition.htm

Salt Institute—Salt and Hypertension http://www.saltinstitute.org/52.html

U.S. Environmental Protection Agency—FAQ: Lead Poisoning
   http://www.epa.gov/region02/faq/lead_p.htm

U.S. Environmental Protection Agency—Fish Advisories http://www.epa.gov/ost/fish

U.S. Department of Health and Human Services and U.S. Environmental Protection
   Agency—What You Need to Know About Mercury in Fish and Shellfish
   http://www.cfsan.fda.gov/~dms/admehg3.html

The Vegetarian Resource Group—Calcium in the Vegan Diet
   http://www.vrg.org/nutrition/calcium.htm

REFERENCES

1. Brody J. A dietary mineral you need and probably didn't know it. *NY Times (Print)* 2004.
2. Massé PG, Dosy J, Tranchant CC, et al. Dietary macro- and micronutrient intakes of nonsupplemented pre- and postmenopausal women with a perspective on menopause associated diseases. *J Hum Nutr Diet*. 2004;17(2):121–132.
3. Valimaki MJ, Laitinen KA, Tahtela RK, et al. The effects of transdermal estrogen therapy on bone mass and turnover in early postmenopausal smokers: a prospective, controlled study. *Am J Obstet Gynecol*. 2003;189(5):1213–1220.

4. Moyad MA. Calcium oxalate kidney stones: another reason to encourage moderate calcium intakes and other dietary changes. *Urol Nurs*. 2003;23(4):310–313.

5. Presne C, Monge M, Bataille P, et al. Randomized trials in the prevention of recurrent calcium stones. *Nephrology* 2003;24(6):303–307.

6. Curham GC. Dietary factors and the risk of incident kidney stones in younger women: nurses' health study II. *Arch Intern Med*. 2004;164(8):885–891.

7. Billings RJ, Berkowitz RJ, Watson G. Teeth *Pediatrics* 2004;113(Suppl 4):1120–1127.

8. Limdi JK, Crampton JR. Hereditary hemochromatosis. *QJM* 2004;97(6):315–324.

SUGGESTED READING

Centers for Disease Control and Prevention. Blood lead levels in residents of homes with elevated lead in tap water—District of Columbia, 2004. *MMWR Morb Mortal Wkly Rep*. 2004;53(12):268–270.

Diaz JH. Is fish consumption safe? *J La State Med Soc*. 2004;156(1):42, 44–49.

Gidlow DA. Lead toxicity. *Occup Med*. 2004;54(2):76–81.

Needleman H. Lead poisoning. *Annu Rev Med*. 2004;55:209–222.

Suzuki Y, Davison KS, Chilibeck PD. Total calcium intake is associated with cortical bone mineral density in a cohort of postmenopausal women not taking estrogen. *J Nutr Health Aging*. 2003;7(5):296–299.

Troost, FJ, Brummer RJM, Dainty JR, et al. Iron supplements inhibit zinc but not copper absorption in vivo in ileostomy subjects. *Am J Clin Nutr*. 2003;78(5):1018.

Yip HK, Li DK, Yau DC. Dental amalgam and human health. *Int Dent J*. 2003;53(6): 464–468.

CHAPTER 7

WATER

OBJECTIVES

Upon completion of the chapter, the reader will be able to:

1 Define homeostasis and give an example of how the body attains it
2 List at least five roles of water in the body
3 Explain how water acts as a solvent during metabolic processes
4 Discuss why the female body contains less water than the male body
5 Explain how we meet our daily need for water and the importance of meeting the need
6 State the recommended daily intake (RDI) for water and list sources
7 Differentiate between water intoxication and water imbalance
8 List symptoms of water dehydration
9 Discuss the difference between hard and soft water
10 Explain which water is best for drinking—tap, bottled, spring, or distilled.

KEY TERMS

Antidiuretic Hormone
    (ADH)
Dehydration
Diuretic

Edema
Extracellular
Homeostasis
Intracellular

Noxious Substance
Potable
Solute

TABLE 7-1   Tissue Water Weight
The following are estimates of percentage of water weight:
Brain 90%
Lungs 90%
Blood 80%
Muscle 80%
Skin 80%
Organs 80%
Fat depots 25%
Bones 22%

A water molecule consists of two hydrogen and one oxygen atoms and in its pure form is a neutral 7pH. It is the only natural substance found in all three states—liquid, solid, and gas. Water is essential for life, with our need for it being second only to oxygen. We can survive about 28 days without food but will be in serious trouble after 3 days without water.

Just as water is abundant on earth, so it is in body tissues. Water is *everywhere* in the human body, with total composition being roughly 45% to 70%. This is more than all other tissues combined. The range may seem large, but is dependent on fat content. The more predominant the fat depots, the less percentage water composition. Women have a lower percentage of water than men, because they usually have more subcutaneous fat deposits, and fat has a lower percentage of water. Table 7-1 estimates water content of body structures.

Our body's water comes from daily food, drink, and metabolic processes. The hydrogen in our food combines with oxygen that we breathe, which creates H_2O

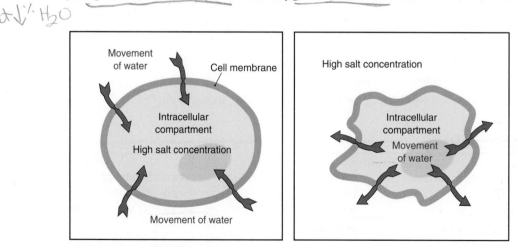

FIGURE 7-1   Flow of water.

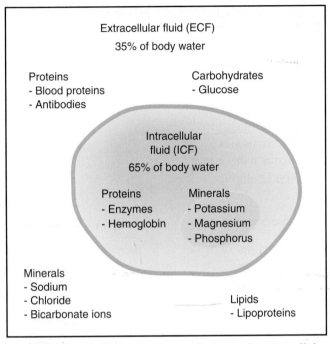

FIGURE 7-2 Contents of intracellular and extracellular compartments.

molecules. Even though our bodies can generate water, it is not enough to sustain life after a few days. We must hydrate ourselves on a daily basis to replenish that which gets lost. Maintaining **homeostasis**, or the proper amount of water for our body is very important because nearly all of our body's chemical reactions depend on water. Fluid within the cells accounts for two thirds of our body's water, and the rest is outside and between cells as blood plasma and lymph. Figure 7-1 illustrates the flow of water between the two compartments, and Figure 7-2 details the contents of intracellular and extracellular water.

🍎 **FOOD FOR THOUGHT 7-1**

Although water covers 326 million cubic miles of the earth's surface, less than 1% is available to drink because the rest is frozen in ice caps and ice bergs or is oceanic salt water. Usable water is found in aquifers, rivers, and fresh water lakes. The amount of water on planet earth is the same as at its creation; water constantly recirculates but cannot be created. It is possible to be drinking the same water dinosaurs drank (www.epa.gov).

MAJOR ROLE OF WATER IN THE HUMAN BODY

Solvent

- Acts as a solvent to make chemical reactions possible
- Removes and dilutes toxic waste
- Is a major transport system
- Builds tissue
- Regulates body temperature
- Cushions delicate tissues
- Moistens mucous membranes
- Maintains blood volume

Water Acts as a Solvent

w/in a cell

One of the main functions of water is to provide the solution for metabolic processes to take place. Water is stored **intracellularly** (65% of body water), where metabolic work takes place, and **extracellularly** (35% of body water), serving as a transport for nutrients and wastes throughout the body.

Water is constantly passes in and out through cell membranes, with the help of the electrically charged minerals of sodium, potassium, and chloride make this possible (see Chapter 6) This is sometimes referred to as a "pumping action" that maintains homeostasis—water balance—within and between our cells.

🍎 **FOOD FOR THOUGHT 7-2**

To give an idea of how much water content is in our bodies, picture 10- or 12-Ga containers lined up. You would think if we were that much water we would slosh when we walked. All that water is within every body cell, neatly encased by cell walls and membranes

---

Water Removes Toxic Waste

Water removes toxic waste, like dissolved flavoring compounds and **noxious substances** that are accidentally ingested. Our bodies must remove the waste even in the absence of fluid intake to keep from being poisoned. Total body water loss comes from two-thirds urine and one-third evaporation through the lungs and skin. Kidneys help accomplish this by producing a minimum of one pint of urine

1/3 lungs + skin - water evaporation
2/3 - urine - water evaporation

each day. We lose approximately 2.5 cups of fluid from normal perspiration and up to 3 Ga or more if exercising for an extended period in a hot climate. It is necessary to drink pure water each day to provide our body with the solution to remove toxins and waste. Think of washing dirt from hands. You would not wash them in soda, juice, or milk as they would all leave more residue to clean.

Water Acts as a Transport System and Maintains Blood Volume

Water not only removes toxic and metabolic waste but also delivers nutrients by way of blood and lymph systems. Our blood constitutes 80% water and about 90% plasma. Plasma carries carbohydrates, proteins, lipids, enzymes, and hormones to all body cells. Lymph fluid carries and mixes extracellular fluid. One of the major functions of lymph fluid is to circulate proteins after they leave the bloodstream.

The body has use for small amounts of carbon dioxide (CO_2) and all excess must be eliminated. Cells expel CO_2 into extracellular fluid, which carries it through the bloodstream to the lungs where it is exhaled.

Water Builds Muscle

Muscle is about 80% water and so it makes sense that to build muscle the body must have water. Muscle holds more water than fat. Men generally have leaner muscle mass than women; therefore, the female body has lower water content than the male body. Less muscle mass and higher body fat ratios equal less water. Obese people have smaller percentages of water because body fat does not hold water.

Water Regulates Body Temperature

Normal body temperature is a dynamic relationship between heat production and heat loss. Water transports heat from one part of the body to another and evaporates from the skin and lungs to control body temperature. Because the body uses water as a coolant, any condition that increases body temperature, such as physical activity or fever, increases the need for water.

Water Cushions and Moistens Delicate Tissues

Water cushions delicate tissues in body structures. Synovial fluid in joints, vitreous fluid in eyes, and fluid in the spinal cord cushions and protects. Water acts as a lubricant to permit movement without friction for our gastrointestinal and respiratory tracts.

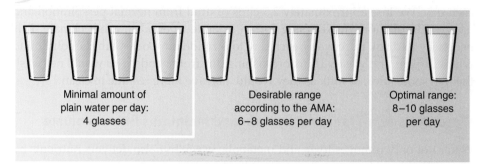

FIGURE 7-3   Recommended water intake. AMA, American Medical Association.

RECOMMENDED DAILY INTAKE

Every day, we lose an average of 10 cups of water through a combination of breathing, urination, and feces elimination. This amount must be replaced daily or the body will be in a state of **dehydration**. At the very least, humans need a little over one quart of water each day just to replenish unavoidable losses in urine, feces, sweat, and expired air. Eight 8-oz. glasses of water per day for the average *inactive* man or woman has been recommended. Figure 7-3 illustrates the amount of recommended daily water intake.

If this amount is more than you usually drink and you suddenly increase the water intake, you will temporarily increase your frequency of urination. Over time, the body will eventually accommodate the increased water intake without any noticeable side effects.

MEETING OUR DAILY REQUIREMENT

We meet our daily water needs through food and beverages and water created from metabolic processes. Approximately 300 mL of water is released as the body metabolizes carbohydrates, proteins, and lipids; this must also be accounted for when meeting water needs. Drinking water and other beverages supplies the body with most of its required daily intake. Caffeinated beverages such as coffee, tea, and colas can function as a **diuretic**, causing the body to lose water, but you still end up with some water available from the beverage for bodily functions. Food for Thought 7-3 identifies water sources in diet.

[handwritten margin notes:]
lose 10 cups/day
needs at least 1 qt. day to replenish
diuretic - any substance that promotes the production of urine. - tea, coffee, colas

> ### 🍎 FOOD FOR THOUGHT 7-3
>
> **SOURCES OF DIETARY WATER**
> One third comes from foods.
> Two thirds come from beverages.

Foods like soup, salads, fruits, and vegetables also supply the body with water. Most foods offer the benefit of some water—even the driest cracker contains almost 3% of water. Fatty foods and those with high sucrose content, however, are not very hydrating, if at all. Food for Thought 7-4 offers advice regarding solutes in beverages.

sucrose - sugar (glucose or fructose)

> ### 🍎 FOOD FOR THOUGHT 7-4
>
> **ALL BEVERAGES ARE NOT EQUAL**
> Juice, soft drinks, and soup all add fluid to the body, but they also add solutes that must be diluted as they enter the bloodstream.

Table 7-2 shows approximate percentage of water content in some common foods.

WATER INTOXICATION

Although water **intoxication** is uncommon, it can occur. It usually happens when the kidneys are not functioning properly and are unable to excrete water as quickly as needed. Symptoms include headache, nausea, and uncoordinated movements with possible progression to unconsciousness, bloating, low body temperature, and seizures. These changes occur because water follows sodium—the excess water dilutes sodium in the blood, causing swelling of cells. This changes the osmotic pressure in tissues as water flows from extracellular fluid into cells. The increase in body fluid can put pressure on the brain, which can lead to seizures or death. This increase also causes the blood volume to drop, which could lead to circulatory shock.

↑ pressure on brain - water intoxication → seizure or death

TABLE 7-2	Percentage of Water in Common Foods
Food	**Water (%)**
Lettuce	98
Celery	96
Watermelon	92
Carrots	90
Milk	88
Oranges	87
Pears	85
Broccoli	85
Apples	84
Peaches	83
Blueberries	80
Beans	79
Eggs	75
Bread	37
Margarine	15
Nuts	5
Crackers	3

WATER DEFICIENCY

Thirst is the first sign of **dehydration**. Everyone experiences mild dehydration on a daily basis—the headachy, vague feeling that something is not right. You might feel heartburn, stomach cramps, low-back pain, or fatigue. If not alleviated, thirst can progress rapidly to weakness, exhaustion, delirium, and in the most extreme case, death. Even if water balance is restored after significant dehydration, kidneys may have been permanently damaged.

Aging affects our body's need and use of water. By the age of 35, all five senses and most organ function begin to diminish. We lose the capability to feel thirsty and our body does not conserve water as efficiently.[1] As a result, the elderly are at risk for dehydration. Infants and children are also at risk of dehydration because their bodies contain more water per pound than the bodies of adults.

Dehydrating factors to consider are as follows:

- Symptoms include thirst, dark-yellow urine, difficulty concentrating, and slight headache.
- Caffeinated beverages affect your hormones that regulate the body's fluid balance, causing more urine production.
- Sugar and salt in fruit juices, soups, and soft drinks increase the concentration of **solutes** in blood. The body's first response is to pull fluid from the cells into the bloodstream to dilute the sugar and salt.
- Nicotine is dehydrating.
- You can lose up to 2 lbs after 3 hours on a plane because of dehydration.

EDEMA/WATER RETENTION

Edema occurs when water from blood plasma flows out of the circulatory system and into the extracellular spaces between the cells. Sometimes the leakage is severe enough to cause the appearance of a fat belly on a starving child. (Lack of protein promotes water retention in the bloodstream.) An example of mild edema would be when you rise in the morning and your fingers feel swollen or blanch at the knuckles when you try to bend them; this is water retention in the joints and is your body's way of conserving water when it is poorly hydrated. Staying well-hydrated can easily reverse mild instances of edema.

ANTIDIURETIC HORMONE AND WATER EXCRETION

An **antidiuretic hormone** (ADH), secreted from the pituitary gland, affects fluid balance by regulating retention and excretion of water through the kidneys. If minerals become too concentrated in any one compartment of the body, they will pull fluid from other compartments to dilute themselves. Here is an example of how it works:

- You eat pizza and find yourself feeling thirsty.
- Sodium from highly salted food accumulates in the extracellular fluid and pulls water from your cells.

- Sensors in the cells signal your brain of the danger in cellular dehydration and you become thirsty.
- You drink until you no longer feel thirsty.
- By drinking more than the cells need, your body will signal the kidneys to make more urine by filtering the excess fluid out of the blood.

The ability of the salt to attract water is the reason why it has been used to clean wounds and preserve meats. It kills bacteria by dehydrating them.

POTABLE WATER

Potable water is that which is fit to drink. The purest, healthiest, and tastiest water may come out of your tap. New water is not created—it is recycled through a continuous process of precipitation, percolation, and evaporation.

Water can be categorized as soft or hard, depending on where it comes from underground and its mineral content. Rainwater and irrigation leach pesticides, herbicides, and fertilizers into the water supply, and so it is important to have your drinking water tested periodically.

Soft Water

- Has a low mineral content
- Comes from sources deep in the ground
- Produces good soapsuds

Hard Water

- Comes from shallow sources and is usually high in calcium and magnesium
- Reduces the sudsing action
- Produces mineral deposits in pipes, tubs, and sinks, and on clothes and dishware

Table 7-3 compares soft and hard water.

STORING WATER

If you have to store water for future use, it is best to store it in a container that has been sterilized with Clorox or soaked in a baking soda solution. Glass

TABLE 7-3   Soft and Hard Water

Soft Water	Hard Water
Low mineral content	High mineral content
Source deep in the ground	Shallow sources
Good sudsing action	Poor sudsing action
Pipes remain clean	Produces mineral deposits in pipes, tubs, and sinks and on clothes and dishware

containers are superior because plastic containers may leach harmful chemicals into the water if exposed to extreme temperatures. Replenish holding containers with new water every few weeks so that bacteria do not grow.

BOTTLED WATER

The U.S. International Bottled Water Association reported yearly profits in excess of $6.4 billion. There are more people buying bottled water than ever imagined 20 years ago, and each year the figures increase. Soda bottlers have ensured their part of the profits by selling water next to their sodas on store shelves. Pepsi bottles Aquafina and Coke bottles Dasani. More than 700 brands of water are offered worldwide. Most bottled water is simply municipal tap water that has been processed for purification and taste.

Environmentalists encourage us to think of the 1.5 million tons of plastic used each year to bottle water. The manufacturing and disposal of plastic bottles release toxic chemicals into the environment that can create climactic change. Food for Thought 7-5 lists common categories of water.

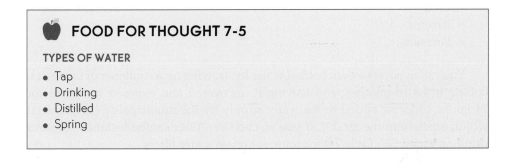

🍎 FOOD FOR THOUGHT 7-5

TYPES OF WATER

- Tap
- Drinking
- Distilled
- Spring

PUBLIC WATER SYSTEMS

protect public health by assuring the safety, efficancy + security

The U.S. Food and Drug Administration (FDA) regulates bottled water, whereas the Environmental Protection Agency (EPA) regulates tap water. The EPA sets safety standards for tap water in the United States, imposing limits on 80 potential contaminants. Although your municipal water supply may meet these limits, it can still make you sick. In 2002, the EPA tested 8,100 of the 55,000 municipal water systems and found that 10% had unsafe levels of lead, which is known to cause permanent neurologic damage. In 2 years, the EPA issued more than 300,000 violations to water systems around the country for failing to test or treat the water properly. Many municipalities failed to notify the public when known contaminants were at higher-than-safe levels. Even if the contaminants in your tap water meet the minimum requirements, "a lot can happen to your water on the way to the tap,"[2] such as:

- It can become laced with pesticides that are washed into rivers and streams.
- It can be affected by chlorine used to disinfect the water reacting with decaying leaves and forming toxic byproducts.
- It can be contaminated by lead from pipes.

HOW SAFE IS YOUR DRINKING WATER?

There can be up to 2,000 contaminants in tap water, including some known poisons. To learn more about your municipal water supply, contact the EPA hotline at 1-800-426-4791 or visit www.epa.gov/safewater/. You can also investigate by inquiring at your public water utility. The following is a list of the five most widespread contaminants:

- Disinfection byproducts
- Turbidity
- Lead
- Arsenic
- Parasites

You can make your own bottled water by drawing up a container of tap water, boiling it for 10 minutes, and leaving it uncovered and exposed to the air for 24 hours. Chlorine added to the water supply by the municipality (to disinfect) will dissipate into the air. Or, if you so choose, a filter can be installed for safer drinking water. See Table 7-4 for information on water filters.

TABLE 7-4	Water Filters		
Purification System	What it Filters	What it Cannot Filter	Comments
Carbon filter	Pesticides Chlorine	Inorganic chemicals Lead Biologic contaminants	
Ceramic filter	Rust Dirt Parasites	Organic pollutants Pesticides	
Ozone	Bacteria Viruses Algae Parasites	Heavy metals Minerals Pesticides	
Ultraviolet (UV) light	Bacteria Viruses	Heavy metals Pesticides Contaminants	
Ion exchange		Everything	Softens Water
Copper-zinc (KDF)	Copper Zinc	Pesticides Organic contaminants	Chemical reaction releases ozone that kills bacteria, chlorine, and heavy metals; works like a magnet
Reverse osmosis	90%–80% heavy metals Bacteria Viruses Organic and inorganic chemicals		Wastes 3–8 Ga of water for every gallon purified
Distillation	Bacteria Viruses Parasites Pathogens Pesticides Herbicides Organic and inorganic chemicals Heavy metals Radioactive contaminants		Uses more electricity than other systems; produces heat when operating Organic chemicals boil at a lower temperature than water and will rise to mix with water vapor—ends up in drinking water

KDF, kinetic degradation fluxion.

DISTILLED WATER

Distilled water is processed to remove all minerals and impurities. It is advisable to keep bottles of distilled water capped when not in use because exposure to air causes impurities to be absorbed by the water. Distilled water is not recommended for drinking; there is speculation that when you drink distilled water, it can attract minerals from your body, depleting them as they are excreted in urine.

SPRING WATER

Spring water comes from a natural spring and contains minerals indigenous to the area. Trace minerals—calcium, magnesium, potassium, phosphorus, copper, and zinc—are sometimes too small to measure. If you want to bottle your own water from a nearby spring, ozonate or disinfect the water before drinking to minimize the possibility of ingesting dangerous bacterium such as *Giardia*.

COUNSELING PATIENTS

The American Dental Association recommends that you always inquire about primary and secondary sources of water on health history forms to identify the amount of fluoride ingested in water. It supports the labeling of bottled water with the fluoride concentration of the product and means of contact.

When determining how much water a patient should consume on a daily basis, consider the following:

- The American Dental Association recommends informing patients that:
  - Home water treatment systems may remove the fluoride in water
  - Bottled water may or may not contain fluoride
- Beverages such as coffee, tea, soda, and alcohol are considered diuretics and actually deplete water stores. If consuming daily, increase water intake accordingly.
- Fruits and vegetables are the food groups that contain high amounts of water.
- Nuts, meats, grains, and fats have some water content, but much lower than that found in fruits and vegetables.
- Assess for xerostomia and salivary flow by having patients chew sugarless gum.
- Teach label reading for hidden sources of sodium.

- Body weight: The more the patient weighs, the more water is needed. Patients should be drinking half their body weight in ounces.
- Age: The very young and old are at greater risk for dehydration. We lose sense of thirst as we age, and preadolescents sweat less than teens and adults, so body temperature rises rapidly during exercise.
- Level of activity and exercise: Patients should sip water every 15 minutes while exercising.
- Weather and climate: Hot climates and fever increase the body's need for water.
- Illness: Fever, diarrhea, and vomiting cause dehydration.
- Pregnancy: Water is needed to support increased blood supply.

Tips for increasing daily water intake are as follows:

- Drink an 8-oz. glass of water with each meal.
- Take a 16-oz. bottle of water when leaving for work and drink it in the car, train, or subway.
- Take a drink of water every time you pass a drinking fountain.
- Drink water while you prepare the evening meal.
- Take a water bottle with you when you exercise.
- Gradually increase the amount you drink to allow your bladder to adjust.
- Fill an empty milk container daily with water and use it to replenish your cup or bottle to keep track of how much you drink.

Putting This Into Practice

Tear out this page and take it with you to your local grocery store. Compare the bottled water available to consumers.

1. What types of bottled water are available?
2. If drinking water is available, is it bottled from another municipality in your state?
3. Call your city or county water utility and ask to speak with a chemist. Find out if your water is soft or hard. Ask which minerals are in the water and in what proportion.

(continued)

4. Write a synopsis of the water purification system and the date of the last treatment center inspection.
5. Write an explanation of the benefits of keeping your body hydrated throughout the day.
6. List some situations that could dehydrate the body.
7. List some benefits to the oral cavity of staying hydrated.

WEB RESOURCES

International Bottled Water Association www.bottledwater.org

The Public Health and Safety Company (certifies products and writes standards to protect food and water) www.nsf.org

U.S. Environmental Protection Agency www.epa.gov

REFERENCES

1. Dupuy N. Mermel VI. Focus on nutrition. St. Louis Mosby, 1995.
2. Schardt D. Water, water, everywhere. *Nutr Action Health Lett* 2000;27:5.

SUGGESTED READING

American Dental Association, House of Delegates. *Policy on bottled water, home water treatment systems and fluoride exposure*. 2002.

Brody J. Must I have another glass of water? Maybe not, a new report says. *NY Times* 2004.

Why we need water. Available at: www.health24.co.za. Accessed October 2003.

CHAPTER 8

DIETARY AND HERBAL SUPPLEMENTS

OBJECTIVES

Upon completion of the chapter, the reader will be able to:

1 Explain what the Dietary Supplement Health and Education Act (DSHEA) means to consumers who use herbal supplements
2 List all the forms of dietary supplements
3 Advise patients as to considerations when purchasing a vitamin/mineral supplement
4 Differentiate between RDA, reference daily intake (RDI), daily value (DV), dietary reference value (DRV), and dietary reference intake (DRI)
5 Discuss why it is difficult to regulate herbal supplement potency

KEY TERMS

Dietary Supplements	RDI	DRV
Herbal Supplements	DV	
RDA	DRI	

In 1994 Congress passed the DSHEA, which defined and set standards for dietary supplements. These were recognized as products that supplement the diet (not *replace sole item of meal* *vitamins minerals*

replace food as a sole item of the meal). As such, **dietary supplements** can be vitamins, amino acids, minerals, herbs, or botanicals and can be in tablet, capsule, powder, tea, softgel, gelcap, or liquid form. This act gave authority to the federal government, more specifically the U.S. Food and Drug Administration (FDA), to ensure the safety of supplements and the accuracy of marketing claims. Food for Thought 8-1 is a synopsis of the 1994 DSHEA law.

🍎 **FOOD FOR THOUGHT 8-1**

1994 DIETARY SUPPLEMENT HEALTH AND EDUCATION ACT
- Product intended to supplement the diet
- Tablet, capsule, powder, softgel, gelcap, or liquid form
- Not to be used as conventional food or as the sole item of a meal
- Labeled as a dietary supplement

Nutritional supplements sold by the multibillion-dollar nutritional supplement industry are regulated by the FDA and considered food supplements—not drugs. Because of this, advertising restrictions are lax and can mislead the unsuspecting consumer to believe anything the supplement purveyors claim. Separating fact from fiction requires careful research and critical thinking because marketers have the ability to persuade the public that supplements can cure all kinds of ills and make other potentially false claims. Fortunately, with the passing of the DSHEA, the federal government was given the authority to ensure our dietary supplements are safe and properly labeled. The FDA has established strict regulatory standards and the new regulations will hold manufacturers accountable for whatever their labels claim. The FDA is able to stop the sale of any dietary supplement that is:

- Adulterated or misbranded
- Marketed with false or unsubstantiated claims that it cures or treats disease
- Posing a significant or unreasonable risk of injury
- Produced in an unclean environment
- Unregulated for potency and stability

False claims

The following is an example of how false claims can be believed by unsuspecting consumers and how the federal government can exercise its power to protect the public from false and misleading claims:

Companies started marketing "Vitamin O" with statements substantiating its function. They claimed that oxygen was vital for life, being the single-most necessary substance for living, and that it fit the definition of a vitamin, which is "a substance found in foods and necessary for life, but not usually manufactured by the body." On May 1, 2000, the Federal Trade Commission charged that the companies made false and unsubstantiated health claims in their advertising for this purported nutritional supplement. The defendants' ads claimed that Vitamin O could treat or prevent serious diseases such as cancer and heart and lung disease by enriching the bloodstream with supplemental oxygen. (Release of the Federal Trade Commission: Marketers of Vitamin "O" Settle FTC Charges of Making False Health Claims; Will Pay $375,000 for Consumer Redress.)

VITAMIN AND MINERAL SUPPLEMENTS

Many people who take vitamin/mineral supplements do so because they think it will keep them healthy, give them more energy, and allow them to live longer. This line of thinking may be giving a false sense of security. According to the UC Berkeley Wellness Guide "There is no evidence that any supplement can prevent colds and infections, reduce fatigue, or improve energy levels." In 2006, a National Institutes of Health (NIH) panel of advisers concluded that "the evidence supporting the benefits and safety of vitamin supplements is limited and inconclusive. Even if you take one, you must still eat a healthy balanced diet."

Most people do not choose foods based on MyPyramid suggestions on a daily basis. As established in Chapter 1, much of our food is bought and eaten at fast food restaurants that offer and serve quick meals high in fat and sodium. The best source of vitamins and minerals are whole foods such as raw fruits and vegetables and whole grains, plus they have added value, which a supplement cannot provide, such as fiber, complex carbohydrates, and phytochemicals that help protect against disease. Individuals who do not have a diet rich in whole foods or routinely choose foods based on MyPyramid could benefit from taking a multivitamin/mineral supplement.

Standing on the supplement aisle at the pharmacy, trying to decide which bottle to purchase can be a daunting proposition. Choices vary in size, price, packaging, and percentage of RDA and one can only wonder if there is a trick to picking the right one or best one. The truth is, several would do the same job. The most important thing to remember when shopping for supplements is to pick one that contains as close to 100% of the recommended dietary allowance (RDA) for each nutrient. There is no need to take more than what is required for one nutrient and less for another. Table 8-1 lists nutrients and suggested DV. Table 8-2 explains specialty vitamins.

TABLE 8-1   Daily Values (DV) of Nutrients

Nutrient	DV	Amount to Look for[a]
B$_1$ Thiamin	1.2 mg	100%
B$_2$ Riboflavin	1.3 mg	100%
B$_3$ Niacin	16 mg	100%; more may cause liver damage
B$_6$	1.7 mg	100%; more may cause reversible nerve damage
B$_{12}$	2.4 µg	100%; people older than 50 yr lack stomach acid needed to extract B$_{12}$ from food—deficiency may cause irreversible nerve damage that can resemble Alzheimer's disease
C	90 mg	250–500 mg will saturate the body's tissues; more than 1,000 mg may cause diarrhea
Folic acid	400 µg	100%; possibly reduces risk for heart disease and colon cancer; reduces the risk of birth defects
A	3,000 IU	3,000 IU retinol; more may increase hip fractures, liver abnormalities, and birth defects; if the label states that vitamin A is from beta-carotene, high doses greater than 15,000 IU may increase risk of lung cancer in smokers
D	400 IU	200 IU for those younger than 50 yr; 400 IU for those older than 50 yr because this age-group gets too little vitamin D from sunshine 600 IU in those older than 70 yr
E	33 IU	Studies did not show a relationship between larger doses and protection against heart disease and stroke; 800 IU and higher may increase risk of dying
K	120 µg	150–250 ideal to reduce hip fractures; interferes with anticoagulant drug therapy
Calcium	1,200 mg	1,000 mg under 50 yr; 1,200 mg in those older than 50 yr; 2,000 mg may increase risk of prostate cancer; a day's worth does not fit in the pill so take a supplement if not eating calcium-rich foods
Iron	18 mg	Men and postmenopausal women need less: 0–8 µg

TABLE 8-1 *(continued)*		
Nutrient	**DV**	**Amount to Look for[a]**
Magnesium	420 mg	Americans get too little from foods; deficiency increases risk for diabetes; more than 350 mg from a supplement may cause diarrhea
Selenium	55 μg	More than 800 μg can cause nails and hair to be brittle; 400 μg is highest safe level
Zinc and copper	0.9 mg	11 mg; 40 mg or higher causes body to lose copper; higher levels of both can depress immune system
Chromium	35 μg	
Iodine		Ignore
Manganese		
Boron Chloride Potassium Biotin pantothenic acid Phosphorus nickel Tin Silicon Vanadium		We get more phosphorus than we need from our diets—too much molybdenum impairs calcium absorption; these are supplied in plenty in our diets and for some, we are not sure why the human body even needs them

[a]Comments taken from "Spin the Bottle," Nutrition Action, 2002.

According to the Mayo Clinic's information on vitamins and supplements, cost is no indicator of the benefit of the supplement and naturally produced vitamins are not nutritionally superior to synthetic vitamins. The body does not recognize the difference between natural and manmade: Both are utilized with the same efficiency and stored and excreted as the body's needs direct. Food for Thought 8-2 contains a kitchen experiment that will help you discover if your body is benefiting from your supplement.

TABLE 8-2　Specialty Vitamins

Vitamin Formula	Distinction
Men's	No more than 9 mg iron
Women's	Premenopausal women 18 mg iron Postmenopausal no more than 9 mg
High potency	At least two thirds of nutrients have 100% DV
Stress	No evidence that the extra B and C vitamins reduce stress or repair the damage
Seniors	Reduced amounts of iron and vitamin K
Energy	The extra B, C, or E vitamins do not give more energy
Antioxidant	Studies do not suggest that vitamins A, C, and E reduce the risk of cancer or heart disease
Lutein	Need at least 14,000 μg to reduce cataracts
Ginseng	Does not boost energy
Ginkgo	Sharper thinking not substantiated

🍎 FOOD FOR THOUGHT 8-2

TRY THIS AT HOME

Place your vitamin, mineral, and herbal supplements in a cup with enough vinegar to cover them. The vinegar represents hydrochloric acid in the stomach and should dissolve your supplements within 30 minutes. If after 30 minutes the supplement is not dissolved, it is probably passing through your system unabsorbed and unutilized.

Consider the following when purchasing a vitamin/mineral supplement:

- Purchase from a place that has a high turnover like Wal-Mart, Kmart, and so on
- Store brands are just as good as the more expensive brands
- Glass amber bottles are best because they do not allow oxygen or light through

- A supplement should dissolve in vinegar within 30 minutes
- Check the expiration date to be sure you have a few months until the bottle expires
- Check for the United States Pharmacopeia (USP) mark—USP is a nongovernmental medical research group; the mark means the supplement has been batch tested for accurate dosage; it does not mean the supplement is safe and effective. Food for Thought 8-3 explains the USP mark.

🍎 FOOD FOR THOUGHT 8-3

USP = UNITED STATES PHARMACOPEIA

Tests supplements for a fee
Means that the supplement dissolves and is made available to the body
Does not mean the supplement is safe or has special benefits

The amount of vitamin or mineral recommended is based on research conducted to discover how much nutrient is needed to perform its specific function. Individual needs differ from small amounts to large quantities. A bell-shaped curve was established for need requirements, and the recommended amount was established so that 95% of the population's needs would be met. Figure 8-1 explains the concept of safe intake.

Reading nutrient charts can get confusing because there are four acronyms that are used interchangeably yet are slightly different in their origination and intended use. Values for each nutrient may vary, depending on which standard is used:

1. **RDA** (recommended dietary allowances): Established by the Food and Nutrition Board of the Institute of Medicine as recommendations—not requirements—designed to meet the needs of healthy people who eat an ample, varied diet. The value is the average amount based on a bell-shaped curve demonstrating the variability of nutrient needs of the population. RDAs were developed during World War II (WWII) by the U.S. National Academy of Sciences in response to investigation of nutritional issues that might affect national defense. The standards were used for nutritional recommendations for armed forces and civilians and considered timely issues such as food rationing.

2. **RDI**: Established by the FDA in 1997 to use in nutritional labeling, based on the highest 1968 RDAs. They are the same as the old United States

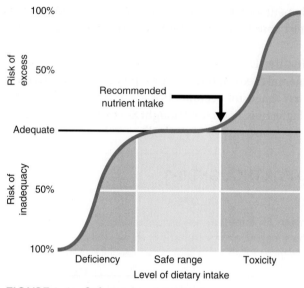

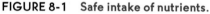

FIGURE 8-1   **Safe intake of nutrients.**

Recommended Daily Allowance (USRDA) and recommend the same level for everyone regardless of age, gender, and other individual differences.

3. **DV**: Same as RDA—the FDA's recommendation on how much of a certain nutrient to aim for on a daily basis. This is the standard seen on food labels.

4. **DRI**: Most recent recommendations established by the Food and Nutrition Board of the Institute of Medicine that takes a more comprehensive approach to determining suggested amount of nutrients. Four different reference values are used to determine levels: RDA, adequate intake, tolerable upper intake level, and estimated average requirement. These values were developed because research justified an increased need for some nutrients to prevent chronic disease. DRIs are used for groups and populations versus individuals. Schools, prisons, hospitals, assisted living facilities use DRIs when planning balanced food menus.

5. **DRV**: British nutrient value recommendations suggested to meet the needs of healthy individuals.

HERBAL SUPPLEMENTS

Dietary supplements known as *herbs* consist of plants or parts of plants to flavor, scent, or add therapeutic value to the diet. Because dietary supplements are regulated by the FDA as foods, they do not always meet the same safety and effectiveness standards as prescription and over-the-counter drugs. As a result, some herbal supplements were found to be contaminated with pesticides, metals, microorganisms, and even some prescription drugs. It is wise to buy from a reputable company with a history of supplying superior products.

Most **herbal supplements** are made from plants, making it difficult to standardize the size of the plant, leaf, or the amount of specific active ingredient. It varies quite a bit from one package to the next, and the part of the plant that contains the active ingredient can differ as well, in regard to the seeds, leaves, bark, stem, and flower. The potency of the active ingredient is affected by climate, soil conditions, quality, preparation, and storage.

🍎 FOOD FOR THOUGHT 8-4

HERBAL MEDICINE

Herbal medicine, also referred to as *phytomedicine, phytotherapy* or *botanical medicine* dates back to medieval times. When the American west was being settled, herbal remedies were all that some doctors had to use. Many of our current prescription drugs have herbal precursors; digitalis is extracted from the foxglove plant, the white willow bark juice contains salic acid which is an ingredient in aspirin

---

🍎 FOOD FOR THOUGHT 8-5

Native American Medicine is herbal based.
   Visit: http://www.powersource.com/cherokee/herbal.html

Why Herbal Supplements?

Dental health care workers need to be aware of their patient's use of herbs when providing oral health care treatment. Many patients will not report taking them unless specifically asked. In a 2006 study conducted with dental patients, the examiners discovered "54% of the participants reported use of herbs. Those using herbs were mostly female, and stated they were less than likely to disclose herbal usage to the practitioner. Of those who reported using herbs, 69% were also on prescription drugs, which could lead to dangerous interactions."[1] A survey conducted in 2002 produced a profile of those most likely to take herbs: educated older women, of average weight, with a healthy lifestyle that included not smoking, exercise, and low-fat diets.[2] The reasons for herbal use are many and varied, so it is important to ensure that herb use is reported on the medical/dental form to better serve our patients. The following are some common reasons for herb usage:

- Failure of traditional medicine to heal
- Lower cost than traditional pharmaceuticals
- Taking control of own health
- Natural and therefore good for the body

This last statement has sometimes been misconstrued to mean that because herbs are natural they are always safe. This is a false assumption because many herbs have been proved to cause serious health problems. Adverse reactions to herbs can be serious. One third of these reactions include heart attacks, liver failure, bleeding, seizures, and death.[3] Of concern to the dental profession is the fact that patients may not be aware that herb consumption should be included on their medical/dental history form. Many herbs interact with traditional medicines, and the health care professional needs to be aware that effects of drugs prescribed could be altered due to herbal medications. Table 8-3 identifies common herbs reported by patients on medical/dental histories.

For various reasons, some patients prefer their dental maladies to be treated with herbs versus traditional medicines and are unaware that some of the herbs can have an effect on their dental treatment. For example, gingko, ginseng, and garlic can prevent blood clotting, causing gingival tissues to bleed freely. Kava kava can enhance the sedative effect of anesthesia. St. John's wort should never be taken with other antidepressants. Long-term use of valerian can increase the amount of anesthesia needed. Ephedra should never be combined with caffeinated beverages because caffeine increases the effects of ephedra. If patients fail to report herb usage, treatment could be compromised, unknowingly to the health care provider. Table 8-4 lists some herbs that are used to treat specific dental conditions.

If a patient reports taking a herb for medicinal treatment or to enhance health, be sure to cross-reference the herb in a table or the Physician's Desk Reference (PDR) Herbal Supplements Index to identify herb–drug interactions. Table 8-5 identifies some of these herb–drug interactions.

TABLE 8-3   Common Herbs Reported on Medical/Dental Histories

If Your Patient Reports Using	For	Be Concerned About
Aloe	Topical skin lotion	Interaction with other drugs: Digoxin Digitalis Thiazide Corticosteroids
Gingko biloba	Improving mental function Improving circulation Tinnitus Vertigo	May cause increased bleeding time Interaction with other drugs: Coumadin ASA NSAIDs Plavix Ticlid
Echinacea	Enhancing immune system Shortens colds and flu	Interaction with other drugs: Cyclosporins Corticosteroids
Ginseng	Increased energy Improving mental function Reducing cholesterol	Headaches Increased bleeding time Agitation Insomnia Hypertension Interactions with insulin, NSAIDs, warfarin
Garlic	Reducing cholesterol Antibiotic Digestive aid Diuretic Expectorant	Blood thinning Interactions with other drugs: Warfarin Ticlopidine ASA Heparin

Continued

TABLE 8-3 *(continued)*

If Your Patient Reports Using	For	Be Concerned About

St. John's wort	Depression
	Uterine cramping
	Fighting infection
		Dry mouth
		Dizziness
		Photosensitivity
		Headache
		Fatigue
		Interactions with other drugs:
		    Warfarin
		    Prozac
		    Zoloft
		    Paxil
		    Tetracycline
		    Cyclosporin
		    Indinavir
		    Digoxin
		    Theophylline

Saw palmetto	Relief from enlarged prostate symptoms and irritable bladder	GI upset
Kava kava	Relaxation Diuretic Improving sleeping habits	Visual and hearing impairment Loss of tongue control Exacerbated Parkinson's symptoms Affected neck muscles that twists head
Valerian	Improving sleeping habits	Headaches Restlessness Increased sedation
Ma-huang (ephedra)	Colds and bronchitis Weight loss	Hypertension Tachycardia Heart palpitations Dizziness Insomnia Agitation Increased effects of caffeine

ASA, aspirin; NSAIDs, nonsteroidal anti-inflammatory drugs.

TABLE 8-4   Herbs Used by Dental Patients

Herb	Dental Use
Aloe, anise, chamomile, eucalyptus, evening primrose, ginseng, golden seal, horsetail, myrrh, peppermint, red clover, rosemary, sage, skull cap, tea tree oil, wintergreen	Soothe inflamed gingival tissues
Anise, clove, parsley, myrrh, rosemary	Treat halitosis
Burdock, cayenne, chickweed, cloves, comfrey, marigold, marjoram, peppermint, wintergreen	Pain relief
Catnip, chamomile, hops, red clover, rockrose, sage, skull cap, wood betony	Pretreatment relaxation
Dandelion, Echinacea, red clover	Root canal treatment
Annato, Shepherd's purse	Reduce bleeding postextraction
Comfrey, lobelia, marigold	Relieve pain and pressure postorthodontic adjustment
Garlic, red clover	Antibiotic
Wintergreen, witch hazel	Astringent/antiseptic
Black cohosh, burdock, comfrey	Relieve muscle cramps in jaw and neck
Cayenne, hops, marjoram, peppermint	Relief from toothache pain
Elderberry, tea tree oil, yarrow	Enhance healing post surgery
Kelp	Maintenance of healthy oral structures
Prickly ash	Increase flow of saliva
Thyme salve mixed with other herbs	Herpetic outbreak
Violet	Soothes aphthous ulcers

TABLE 8-5 Herbal/Supplements and Drug Interactions

Herbal Supplement	Combined With Prescription	Effect
Alfalfa	Antacids	Mucosal irritation
Caffeine	Ciproflaxacin, enoxacin	Inhibits metabolism of caffeine, tremors, tachycardia
	Cardiac medications	Increases blood pressure
Chamomile	Anticoagulants	Increased bleeding
	CNS depressants	Increased sedative effect
Capsicum	Antacids	Mucosal irritation
	Antihypertensives	Stimulates sympathetic nerve activity
Celery	Diuretic	Increased urination
	Anticoagulant	Increased bleeding
	CNS depressants	Increased sedative effect
	Diabetic medications	Low blood sugar
Cloves	Anticoagulants	Increased bleeding
Dandelion	Diuretics	Increased urination
Dong quai	Anticoagulants	Increased bleeding
	Tamoxifen	Decreased effect
Echinacea	Anabolic steroids	Liver toxicity
	Cyclosporin	Decreased effects
Ephedrine (Ma Huang)	Cardiac medications	Irregular heartbeat, stroke, and blood pressure
		Seizures
	Antidepressants	Increased bleeding
	Anticoagulants	
Eucalyptus	Antacids	Mucosal irritation
Evening primrose	Antiepileptic	Decreased effect
Feverfew	Anticoagulants	Increased bleeding
	Migraine medications	Increased blood pressure and heart rate
Garlic	Anticoagulants	Increased bleeding
	Cholesterol drugs	Decreased cholesterol
	Diabetic medications	Decreased blood sugar levels

TABLE 8-5 *(continued)*

Herbal Supplement	Combined With Prescription	Effect
Ginger	Hypertensive drugs	Irregular heart beat
	Diabetic medications	Decreased blood sugar levels
	Anticoagulants	Increased bleeding
Gingko biloba	Anticoagulants	Prolonged bleeding
Ginseng	Digoxin	Increased blood pressure, irregular heart beat
		Reduced blood coagulation
	Anticoagulants	Altered glucose concentrations
	Insulin	Increased sedative effect
	Antidepressants	
Goldenseal	β Blockers	Increased blood pressure
	Diabetic medications	Electrolyte imbalance
	Diuretics	Increased urination
Guarana	Stimulants	Insomnia, trembling, anxiety, heart palpitations
Horseradish	Thyroid medications	Altered thyroid activity
Kava-kava	Alcohol	CNS overload
	Barbiturates	CNS overload
Kelp	Thyroid medications	Iodine interferes with thyroid replacement
Licorice	Antihypertensives	Decreases urination
	Anticoagulants	Inhibits platelet activity
	Steroids	Increased effects of steroids
	Oral contraceptives	Hypertension, edema, hypokalemia
Myrrh	Thyroid medications	Altered thyroid hormone activity
Parsley	Antacids	Mucosal irritation
Red clover	Anticoagulants	Increased bleeding
Saw-palmetto	Hormones	Increases estrogen and decreases androgenic hormones

Continued

TABLE 8-5 *(continued)*		
Herbal Supplement	**Combined With Prescription**	**Effect**
St. John's wort	HIV protease inhibitors	Loss of HIV suppression
	Cyclosporins	Transplant rejection
	Anticonvulsants	Increased chance of seizures
	Oral contraceptives	Contraceptive failure
	Dexatrim	Increased blood pressure
Valerian	Alcohol	Reduces effect of alcohol
	CNS depressants	Increased sedation
Willow bark	Anticoagulants	Increased bleeding
Zinc	Cyclosporin	Opposite effect

CNS, central nervous system; HIV, human immunodeficiency syndrome.

COUNSELING PATIENTS

It is strongly recommended that before taking herbs, you consult with your physician or a professional trained in herb usage. The following suggestions about taking herbal supplements have been taken from Medfacts, a website supported by the National Jewish Medical and Research Center:

1. Research a herbal supplement before taking it.
2. Do not assume a product is safe or effective.
3. Although touted as natural and safe, herbs act as drugs but may lack scientific study.
4. Follow guidelines for dosages and length of time for which the herb can be safely taken.
5. Buy herbs from reliable sources. Labels should include ingredient list, precautions, manufacturer's name and address, batch or lot number, manufacture date, expiration date, and dosage information.
6. Introduce herbs one at a time to monitor effectiveness and side effects. Using multiple herbal supplements puts you at a greater risk for possible adverse reactions.
7. Do not give herbs to infants or young children.
8. Do not take herbs if you are pregnant, nursing, or planning a pregnancy.
9. Use extreme caution with herbs purchased in other countries or through mail order.
10. Herbs can be part of an overall health maintenance program. Before taking, investigate a product thoroughly.[4]

Putting This Into Practice

Your client is a 28-year-old man with a 3-year history of human immunodeficiency virus (HIV). His medical/dental history indicates use of prescription drugs and herbs. He is taking the usual protease inhibitors (indinivir) prescribed by his physician and self-medicates with St. John's wort to relieve mild depression. Upon oral examination, you note red and edematous gingival tissues that bleed freely upon probing, slow-acting salivary glands, and light retentive plaque.

1. Explain to your client the interaction of indinivir and St. John's wort.
2. What other oral symptoms are caused by St. John's wort that could have an overall effect on active disease?
3. What recommendations might the dentist make to this client to improve his oral health?

WEB RESOURCES

USDA Dietary Supplements http://fnic.nal.usda.gov/nal_display/index.php?info_center= 4&tax_level=2&tax_subject=274&topic_id=1331

Food and Drug Administration Guide on Herbs http://vm.cfsan.fda.gov/~dms/fdsupp.html

http://www.nal.usda.gov/fnic/etext/000015.html

http://vm.cfsan.fda.gov/~dms/supplmnt.html

General Information on Herbal Supplements
http://www.nlm.nih.gov/medlineplus/herbalmedicine.html

http://www.nutritional-supplement-info.com/

http://www.nutritional-supplement-guide.com/html/herbalsupplements.html

http://www.herbmed.org/

http://www.mskcc.org/mskcc/html/11570.cfm

http://www.citizen.org/hrg/drugs/articles.cfm?ID=5195

http://healthlink.mcw.edu/article/964721794.html

Information on Herb and Drug Interactions http://www.everybody.co.nz/otc/herbals.html

Information on Herbs Contraindicated During Pregnancy and Lactation
http://www.marchofdimes.com/professionals/681_1815.asp

http://www.marchofdimes.com/pnhec/159_529.asp

Information on Herbs—National Jewish Hospital http://www.nationaljewish.org

Information on Herbs—Mayo Clinic http://www.cnn.com/HEALTH/library/NU/00205.html

Information on Side Effects, Warnings, and Drug Interactions

  http://www.consumerlab.com/recalls.asp http://www.personalhealthzone.com/herbsafety.html

http://www.consumersunion.org/pub/core_product_safety/000285.html

http://www.hon.ch/News/HSN/511204.html

http://www.tufts-health.com/RxIQ/RxIQ.php?sec=vitaherb&content=vitamins

http://nccam.nih.gov/health/supplement-safety

http://www.hc-sc.gc.ca/english/protection/warnings/2002/2002_46e.htm

REFERENCES

1. Tam KK, Gadbury-Amyot CCCobb CM, et al. Differences between herbal and non herbal users in dental practice. *J Dent Hyg* 2006;80(1):10.
2. Biron C. Herbs: efficacy, adverse reactions, and drug interactions. *RDH* 2004;64–66:92.
3. Schardt D. Are your supplements safe? **Nutr Action Healthletter** 2003;30:3–7.
4. National Jewish Medical and Research Center, Medfacts. *Using herbal supplements wisely*. Available at: www.nationaljewish.org. Accessed November 2008.

SUGGESTED READING

Abebe W. Herbal supplements: any relevance to dental practice? *NY State Dent J* 2002; 68(10):20–30.

Abebe W. An overview of herbal supplement utilization with particular emphasis on possible interactions with dental drugs and oral manifestations. *J Dent Hyg* 2003;77(1):37–46.

Council for Responsible Nutrition. *Historical comparison of RDIs, RDAs and DRI, 1968 to present*. Washington, DC, 2001.

Danner V. *The natural life*. Accessed on April 2001.

Dietary Supplement Bureau. *How dietary supplements are regulated*. Available at: www.supplementinfo.org. Accessed October 2003.

Duke J. *A guide to herbal alternatives. Herbs for health*. November/December 1997.

Genger T. Spin the bottle. *Nutr Act Health lett* 2003.

National Center for Complimentary and Alternative Medicine, National Institute of Health. *Herbal supplements; consider safety too*. Bethesda, MD, 2003.

Office of Dietary Supplements, National Institute of Health. What are dietary supplements. 2003.

Parsa-Stay F. *The complete book of dental remedies*. Garden City Park: Avery Publishing Group; 1996.

Sherman R. Herbal supplements: implications for dentistry. Presented at the *Hawaiian Dental Forum*. Honolulu, 2003.

Spolarich AE, Andrews L. An examination of the bleeding complications associated with herbal supplements, antiplatelet and anticoagulant medications. *J Dent Hyg* 2007; 81(3):67.

RELATIONSHIP OF NUTRITION TO ORAL DISEASE

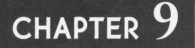

CHAPTER 9

DIET AND DENTAL CARIES

OBJECTIVES

Upon completion of this chapter, the reader will be able to:

1 Understand the relationship between diet and dental caries
2 Discuss the caries process and factors that can decrease caries risk
3 Know the difference between sugar alcohols and synthetic sweeteners
4 Explain how host factors can increase or decrease caries risk
5 Counsel patients on ways to prevent dental caries by making better food choices
6 Recognize oral symptoms of Early Childhood Caries
7 Discuss the benefits of having ample saliva and understand concerns of xerostomia
8 Name the bacteria most responsible for metabolizing carbohydrates and identify various acids created in the process
9 Identify groups most at risk for dental caries

KEY TERMS

Acid Production	Caries Risk	Critical pH 5.5
Calcium	Cariogenic	Early Childhood Caries
Caries Equation	Cariostatic	(ECC)

Fluoride

Host Factors

Lactic Acid

Lactobacillus

Neutral pH 7.0

Phosphate

Phosphoric Acid

Plaque Fluid

Remineralize

Retentive Factor

Salivary Gland Hypofunction

Secretory Leukocyte Protease Inhibitor (SLPI)

Starch

Streptococcus mutans

Sugar

Sodium Bicarbonate

Sugar Alcohol

Synthetic Sweetener

Xylitol

The relationship of diet and dental caries has been well established: frequent consumption of carbohydrates can have a detrimental effect on teeth, which supports the **caries equation** of bacteria + carbohydrate = acid demineralization (Figure 9-1). However over the last 2 decades, sugar (carbohydrate) consumption in the United States has increased steadily, whereas the incidence of dental caries has decreased. Although there is a scientifically established cause and effect relationship, other host factors can water down the strength of the formula. Even with frequent consumption of carbohydrates, by exposing developing and erupted teeth to fluoride, placing sealants, practicing better oral hygiene, and having ample saliva, the caries risk is reduced.

If asked, many patients will say that "sugar" gives you cavities. This is not completely accurate, as all sugars are not the same—some are worse than others. All carbohydrates can demineralize tooth enamel, and **sugar**—or, rather, sucrose—is only one of many sugars. Even though a potato chip does not in any way resemble a piece of sweet candy, it can actually be more detrimental to tooth enamel than a teaspoon of sugar. That is because a potato chip is a "cooked starch," which is a form of carbohydrate. Salivary amylase breaks down the **starch** to a

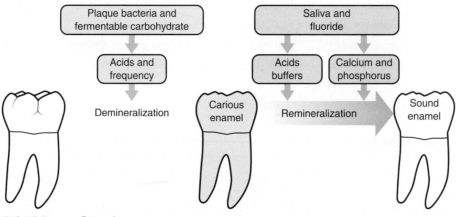

FIGURE 9-1   Dental caries equation.

disaccharide which is metabolized by plaque bacteria, resulting in acid production for as long as the potato chip remains in the mouth. Think back to the last time you ate a potato chips, piece of bread, rice, or cracker. It gets stuck on your teeth and hangs around longer than a piece of hard candy. Then imagine a piece of bread spread with sweet jelly stuck between your teeth. That combination of a starch with sweet is perhaps the most detrimental of all food choices for your teeth. So yes, sugar does cause dental caries, but so do other carbohydrates.

🍎 FOOD FOR THOUGHT 9-1

Sweetness is the only taste a human is born craving. Scientists state that the sense of taste was used to determine if plants and animals were safe to eat—sweet meant safe and bitter unsafe.

🍎 FOOD FOR THOUGHT 9-2

Evidence of sugar consumption appears as early as 2600 BC in Egyptian tomb drawings depicting beekeepers harvesting honey for the privileged class.

🍎 FOOD FOR THOUGHT 9-3

According to the World Health Organization, the average American consumes a little less than 40 lb of sugar per year.

FAMOUS VIPEHOLM STUDY

Much of what we currently know about the relationship between sugar and dental caries was discovered as a result of a study conducted from 1945 to 1953, involving 436 residents at a mental institution in Vipeholm, Sweden. At that time, dental health in Scandinavia was very poor with 83% of 3-year-olds having evidence of dental caries. The Dental Institute in Stockholm made the decision to conduct a clinical trial, seeking definite answers to questions about the relationship linking sugar to dental caries—especially if form of sugar and frequency of eating sugar had any effect on dental caries. Residents were divided into three different groups receiving varying amounts and forms of sugar, either with their regular meals or between meals as snacks.[1]

- All groups received the basal diet (no simple sugars).
- First group ate the basal diet with 300 g of additional sugar in solution during meals.
- Second group ate the basal diet with an additional 50 g of sugar in bread with their meals.
- Third group ate the basal diet with in-between-meal snacks of toffee and candy consisting of a small amount of sugar.

The third group, with the in-between-meal sugared snacks reported the highest caries rate. On the basis of these 8 years of study, it was determined that:

1. Frequency of sugar consumed is the prime factor in caries activity.
2. Form and composition of sweets is important: Foods that stayed in the oral cavity and took longer to clear than liquids increased the rate of caries.
3. Quantity of sugar eaten is not of great importance: An increase from 30 to 330 g per day caused little increase in caries production.
4. Sugar exerts caries-promoting effects locally on tooth surfaces.

FACTORS OF CARIES DEVELOPMENT

There are six factors that determine the caries susceptibility of a tooth:

- Presence of specific bacteria (strep mutans and lactobacillus)
- Susceptible tooth structure
- Carbohydrates in the diet
- Absence of fluoride
- Salivary gland hypofunction (SGH)
- Poor oral hygiene

Evaluation of these six factors, which vary widely from patient to patient, help determine a patient's risk for dental caries. Specific bacteria, carbohydrate consumption and dry mouth all contribute to enamel demineralization, whereas calcium and phosphorous in saliva, professional fluoride application, and use of fluoridated toothpaste on a daily basis will remineralize enamel. Focusing on factors that remineralize enamel will help offset detrimental effects of carbohydrates in the diet.

Bacteria Responsible for Formation of Dental Caries

Streptococcus mutans and *Lactobacillus* are just 2 of more than 500 bacteria found living in dental plaque and are the main bacteria involved in caries formation. The presence of *S. mutans* is needed to initiate pit and fissure, smooth surface, and root surface decay. *S. mutans* starts the process and takes it to the enamodentin junction, where *Lactobacillus* takes over, extending the lesion into the dentin.

Tooth Structure

Posterior molars with shallow grooves are less susceptible to dental caries because they do not retain plaque and food as do molars with very deep grooves. Teeth with deeper grooves retain plaque and food because toothbrush bristles cannot reach to the depth during daily cleaning. Teeth that are rotated or crowded offer protected areas for plaque to grow and are not cleansed by chewing action or quick toothbrushing. The action of chewing has a cleansing effect on teeth that are all in alignment and with shallow grooves.

Host resistance to caries

Generally, a good gene pool and good maternal nutrition will make the difference between carious and caries-free teeth. **Host** factors that reduce caries risk are as follows:

- Teeth with shallow anatomy (pits and fissures)
- Straight teeth in alignment
- Good preeruptive nutrition (certain nutrient deficiencies during fetal development can cause crowded or rotated teeth)
- Well mineralized newly erupted teeth

Cariogenic Properties of Carbohydrates

Factors that determine cariogenicity of the diet are as follows:

1. Physical form of food—liquids clear the oral cavity twice as fast as solid foods and sticky foods hang around the longest.
2. Frequency of eating events—an eating event (snack) is when a carbohydrate food or beverage is consumed 20 minutes on either side of a meal. Snacks are separate opportunities for bacteria to feed and produce acid.
3. Sequence in which foods are eaten—the sequence of foods eaten can minimize effects of acid attack.

4. Fats and proteins eaten in the meal can lay a protective fatty coating on teeth, protecting them from sugars eaten later.
5. Consuming dairy products keeps the saliva rich in calcium and phosphorus, offering the benefit of remineralization.
6. Cheese eaten after a sugar prevents the pH from dropping below 5.5.

Sticky foods such as caramels, jellybeans, gumdrops, and other chewy candies are the foods usually perceived as being most **cariogenic**. The truth, however, is that cookies, crackers, and potato chips are more cariogenic because they are retained longer in the mouth, which means teeth have longer exposure to acid, as the bacteria metabolize the carbohydrate. Aside from the **retentive factor**, starch is the least cariogenic of carbohydrates because it is such a large molecule and must be broken down before it can diffuse through plaque. However, it is still cariogenic because of its more retentive consistency. Consuming foods containing both starch and sugar may be more cariogenic than those with just simple sugars, because starch and sugar together hang around longer, giving bacteria a longer time to produce acid from the readily available sugar. The following are some facts about cariogenic properties of carbohydrates:

- Monosaccharides and disaccharides are the most cariogenic carbohydrates (simple sugars).
- Sucrose is the most cariogenic of all carbohydrates.
- Starch is the least cariogenic carbohydrate.
- Starch eaten with sucrose (e.g., toast with jelly) is more cariogenic that either one alone because starchy foods stick to the teeth longer.
- Natural sugars such as honey, molasses, and raw sugar (turbinado) are just as cariogenic as refined sugars.
- Corn syrups added to foods are just as cariogenic as refined sugars.
- Honey may be more cariogenic because of its thick and sticky properties.
- Powdered sugar is more cariogenic than granulated sugar because it is concentrated and fine.
- Fruits and vegetables and their juices are not as cariogenic as sucrose because of water dilution.
- A food that is 80% sucrose may not be any more harmful than one that is 40% sucrose.

Acidic enamel demineralization

All foods and beverages that contain carbohydrates have the potential to cause dental caries. Plaque bacteria feed on carbohydrates and produce acid that can demineralize enamel. Some foods are naturally acidic and erode enamel.[1] If acid byproducts from metabolized carbohydrates or acidic foods drop the **normally basic 7 pH** of the mouth below the **critical pH level of 5.5**, enamel demineralization begins. Demineralized enamel appears as a rough parchment-white spot on the tooth, usually on the gingival 1/3 where plaque accumulates. There are five different acids that are created when carbohydrates are metabolized by bacteria.

1. Lactic—most abundant
2. Formic
3. Proprionic
4. Acetic
5. Buturic

The drop in pH starts within seconds and can become critical in about 5 minutes. The demineralization continues until the pH of the mouth is returned to 7.0 (basic).

Fluoride

If a patient reports heavy consumption of sugar, presence of **fluoride** will reduce its detrimental effect on teeth.[2] Ingestion of fluoride, either in food or water, will increase the fluoride content of saliva, making it available to strengthen and **remineralize** enamel. Salivary fluoride levels are elevated for up to 3 hours after brushing with fluoridated toothpaste, bathing teeth, and remineralizing enamel. Fluoride can also accumulate in **plaque fluid**, offering protective factors adjacent to enamel surfaces.[3,4]

Saliva

After fluoride, adequate **saliva** is the number one protector of teeth.[3–5] Saliva is saturated with calcium, phosphate, sodium bicarbonate, and proteins. **Calcium** and **phosphate** are components of enamel and can repair demineralized areas. **Sodium bicarbonate** (baking soda) has a high pH and can neutralize acids in the mouth that demineralize enamel. Saliva also "washes" or clears solid and liquid foods from the oral cavity, reducing the amount of time bacteria can feed on carbohydrates and manufacture acid. Saliva dilutes acids and carries them out with the flow of saliva. A multifunction protein in saliva called **secretory leukocyte protease inhibitor** (**SLPI**) has antiviral, bacterial, and fungal properties that reduce and render ineffective caries causing bacteria in plaque.[5] Eating crunchy or chewy foods will increase salivation and are therefore most desirable. Consuming at least one chewy or crunchy food at each meal is recommended.

Salivary Factors

- Physical
  - Saliva rinses teeth free of food particles, especially if forced around and in between teeth.
  - Viscous saliva is not as effective as more fluid saliva at rinsing teeth.
  - If a client has an abundance of saliva, food clears the oral cavity faster and so pH will return to 7.0 more quickly.
- Chemical
  - Saliva has sodium bicarbonate, which buffers acid at the plaque/enamel interface.
  - Saliva has calcium and phosphorus, which remineralizes enamel.
  - A protein called "sialin" in saliva reduces the amount of pH drops and also helps the oral pH return to 7.0 quicker.
  - As saliva flow is stimulated (by chewing firm foods) and the amount of saliva increases, there is an increase of remineralizing, buffering, and antibacterial components.
- Antibacterial
  - Mucins in saliva trap bacteria and remove it with normal swallowing patterns.
  - Proteins in saliva are antibacterial.

Oral Hygiene

The motivation and ability to remove bacterial plaque plays a major role in keeping teeth caries free. To increase the number of bacteria in the mouth, plaque must be left on the teeth and carbohydrates must be eaten. When carbohydrates are eaten, plaque becomes stickier and more food is stored to support more bacteria, providing more places for bacteria to exist. Scrupulous home care that removes bacterial plaque on a daily basis eliminates that component in the caries equation.

Plaque, Saliva, and Acid Facts

- Plaque holds bacteria close to the enamel.
- When carbohydrates are eaten, they diffuse through the plaque and are metabolized by plaque bacteria.
- The end product is acid.
- **Lactic acid** production causes the pH at the plaque/enamel interface to drop from 7.0 to less than 5.5 within seconds.

- If plaque is immature and not very thick, saliva may penetrate plaque and buffer the acid.
- As plaque thickens, saliva cannot buffer acid as easily.
- Acid production continues until carbohydrates are cleared from the mouth.
- Demineralization stops when carbohydrates are cleared.
- Once food is cleared and acid production stops, remineralization can begin.
- If the patient uses fluoridated toothpaste or drinks fluoridated water, the remineralized area may be stronger than before acid attack.

EARLY CHILDHOOD CARIES

Figures 9-2 through 9-6 show varying forms of ECC, also known as "bottle-mouth" caries, in children of different ages.

In 1994, the Centers for Disease Control (CDC) changed the name of bottle-mouth caries to **Early Childhood Caries** (ECC), declaring the former name to be too misleading. ECC can be diagnosed if decay is present on one or more smooth surfaces, but is usually seen as extensive decay of all deciduous teeth, in children aged 5 years or younger.[6] Sometimes the mandibular anterior teeth are spared because they are protected by the tongue and saliva. It was believed to occur when a child was put to bed with a bottle of milk or sweetened drink, hence the name "bottle-mouth" caries, but recent studies show that children with ECC have more *S. mutans* bacteria in their mouths than children without caries. Bacteria feed on

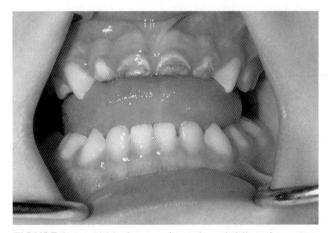

FIGURE 9-2 Mild form of early childhood caries.
(Courtesy of Dr. William Chambers, Asheville, NC.)

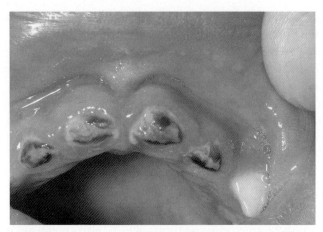

FIGURE 9-3   Early childhood caries in an 18-month-old child. (Courtesy of Dr. William Chambers, Asheville, NC.)

the milk (carbohydrate), produce acid, and demineralize enamel. Children quit sucking when they fall asleep, allowing whatever is in the bottle—formula, milk, juice, breast milk—to pool around teeth, thus beginning the demineralization process. Because saliva production slows during sleep, the protective factors of saliva are not available. The American Academy of Pediatric Dentists recognizes ECC as an epidemic, especially in populations of ethnic minorities. There have been reports that breastfeeding can cause dental caries, but according to studies

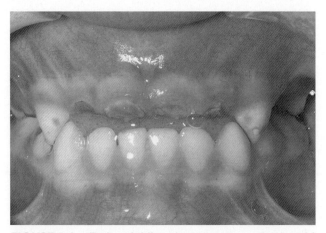

FIGURE 9-4   Early childhood caries in a 2-year-old child. (Courtesy of Dr. William Chambers, Asheville, NC.)

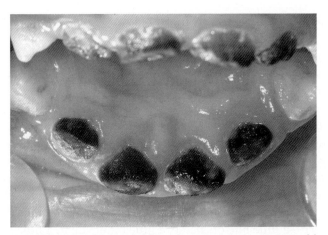

FIGURE 9-5   Early childhood caries in a 3-year-old child. (Courtesy of Dr. William Chambers, Asheville, NC.)

conducted by the National Institute of Dental and Craniofacial Research, breastfed children are less likely to develop this disease than those who are fed by bottle. ECC can be prevented if the child is weaned from the bottle by around 9 months old or if they are fed before being put to bed. More importantly, however, daily removal of bacterial plaque by brushing or wiping contributes more to preventing ECC. It is suggested to fill the bottle with plain water if a child must be put to bed with a bottle.

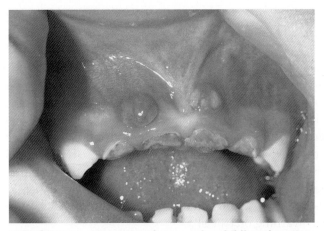

FIGURE 9-6   Abscesses from early childhood caries. (Courtesy of Dr. William Chambers, Asheville, NC.)

CARIOSTATIC FOODS

Cariostatic foods are those that do not contribute to initiation of demineralization or continue the caries process. Some foods and nutrients have cariostatic properties and can actually help prevent dental caries.

- Fats do not lower oral pH to an acidic level and can actually increase the pH after consuming carbohydrates. Fats in the meal should be eaten before sugary dessert.
- Proteins elevate salivary urea, which buffers acid. It has been found that if high-protein foods are eaten after a carbohydrate, the pH returns to 7.0 more quickly. The sequence in which foods are eaten may make a difference—a little bite of cheese, a little bit of sugar, a little bite of cheese, and so on. Protein in the meal, like fats, should be eaten before sugary dessert.
- Phosphates also buffer acid. In animal studies where phosphates were added to the diet along with sugar, caries did not occur, but the cariostatic activity of phosphate had no lasting effect as fluoride did.
- Fluoride has protective factors that can continue well after the meal has been eaten. Fluoride is naturally occurring in small quantities in some foods such as tea and seafood. The fluoride from the food, water, or beverage makes its way to the saliva, where it bathes the teeth and infiltrates plaque, protecting teeth from acid attacks. Fluoride has both antibacterial and antiplaque capabilities.

SUGAR SUBSTITUTES

Sugar substitutes are a multimillion-dollar industry. **Synthetic sweeteners** like saccharine, aspartame, and sugar alcohols are used in many foods to reduce the caries-causing potential of the sugar.[7] Both synthetic sweeteners and sugar alcohols are noncariogenic, but only the synthetic sweeteners are noncaloric.

Placed next to regular table sugar, **sugar alcohols** are visually the same, but they are different in that they do not raise blood glucose levels as table sugar does. Sugar alcohols are made by adding hydrogen atoms to sugar. When sugar alcohol enters the intestines, it can cause cramping, bloating, and diarrhea. Because of this, the U.S. Food and Drug Administration (FDA) mandates that manufacturers place a laxative effect warning on labels.

Examples of Sugar Alcohols

- **Xylitol** is the alcohol form of xylose and is the most desirable of all sugar substitutes for two reasons:
  1. Bacterial plaque does not metabolize xylitol.
  2. Xylitol has the ability to reduce salivary *S. mutans* in the mouth.[2]

University of Michigan researchers found that school children who chewed gum with xylitol for 5 minutes, three to five times a day, not only reduced caries but also remineralized incipient lesions.[8] Xylitol occurs naturally in straw, corncobs, fruit, vegetables, cereals, mushrooms, and some seaweed and is made from birch tree chips in Europe and corn stalks in the United States. It has the same sweetness as sucrose.

- Sorbitol is an alcohol form of sucrose made by adding hydrogen to glucose. Research concludes that chewing gum with sorbitol after eating significantly reduced incidence of dental caries.[9] Sorbitol occurs naturally in fruits and vegetables and is manufactured from corn syrup.
- Maltitol is the alcohol form of mannose and naturally occurs in pineapples, olives, asparagus, sweet potatoes, and carrots. It is extracted from seaweed for use in manufacturing.

Lesser Known Sugar Alcohols

- Mannitol
- Lactitol
- Isomalt
- Erythritol

Synthetic Sweeteners

The FDA approves sugar substitutes for use in foods and beverages after extensive animal studies have been conducted to determine if it is safe for human consumption. The most commonly used sweeteners are aspartame, saccharin, and sucralose.

- Aspartame (NutraSweet, Equal, or Nutra Taste) is 180 times sweeter than sucrose and is used by more than 100 million people globally. Aspartame is made of aspartic acid and the amino acid phenylalanine. It is toxic to those with phenylketonuria (PKU). Many people claim to have adverse reactions—anywhere from forgetfulness or brain fog to seizures and migraines. Research has found these claims to be unfounded. Neotame is made of the same ingredients as aspartame but is more stable and is not metabolized by the body like aspartame.

- Saccharin (Sweet 'N Low) is 300 times sweeter than sucrose and was at one time considered unsafe. In 1977, the FDA tried to ban saccharin because animal studies showed that it caused cancer of the bladder, the reproductive organs, and other vital organs. A warning notice was put on Sweet 'N Low packets and on some food products containing saccharin. In the late 1990s, the Calorie Control Council had Congress reverse the adverse warning when they proved humans and rats do not develop cancer in the same manner. Research on saccharin continues. As recently as 2002, a study proved that consumers who drank more than two diet drinks per day or used more than six packets of saccharin daily had a small increased chance of developing bladder cancer.[10]
- Sucralose (Splenda) is the only sugar substitute made from sugar and is made by chlorinating sucrose. It remains stable at high temperatures, making it an ideal substitute for sugar in recipes. Users report no bitter aftertaste as with saccharin and aspartame. Sucralose is produced by chemically changing the structure of sugar molecules by substituting three chlorine atoms for three hydroxyl groups. With this chemical change, the body is unable to burn sucralose for energy. In 1976, Diet RC Cola was the first product manufactured with Splenda. Although sucralose has thus far passed all safety tests and animal studies, reported adverse effects include enlarged kidney and liver.

Many people report incompatibility with most of the sugar substitutes, the major complaints being headaches and diarrhea. This is important to know when recommending suggestions for making better food and beverage choices. Diabetic patients have no choice but to use synthetic sweeteners. If your patient is diabetic and is not amenable to using sugar substitutes, the following can be suggested as alternatives:

- Stevia (Sweet Leaf and Honey Leaf) is a plant derivative from South America. Like artificial sweeteners, stevia is not metabolized by the human body like sugar. Animal studies indicated that stevia caused infertility, so as a result, the FDA, the World Health Organization, and Canadian and European food watchdogs warn that stevia should not be used to sweeten food and beverages.[10] Currently, it is sold as a supplement and can be purchased in health food stores as an alternative to saccharine, aspartame, and sucralose.

- Sucanet is whole cane sugar with water removed.
- Fruit juice.

GROUPS AT RISK FOR DENTAL CARIES

Not all clients are in need of diet counseling for dental caries, so it is imperative to identify those groups with the highest risk. An evaluation for **caries risk** should be completed on every new and returning patient of any age to formulate the best plan for preventive treatment. Caries risk assessment tools determine previous experience with caries, source and amount of fluoride, meal/snacking habits, socioeconomic status, amount of bacterial plaque, nature of saliva, and frequency of dental visits.

Patients of all ages and socioeconomic status can develop dental caries, but those considered most at risk are children and elderly.[11]

🍎 FOOD FOR THOUGHT 9-4

GROUPS AT RISK FOR DENTAL CARIES

- Those with a high-carbohydrate diet
- Children/adolescents
- Elderly
- Those with past experience with dental caries
- People with xerostomia
- Those who have inadequate fluoride intake
- People with poor oral hygiene practices

An eating event refers to an exposure to carbohydrate 20 to 30 minutes before or after a meal. Figure 9-7 demonstrates caries from frequent exposure to dental caries. If we take what we learned from the Vipeholm study, frequency of eating carbohydrates has a detrimental effect on teeth. Children average seven eating events in a day, most of which contain foods with added sugar. People who have more than three to five exposures per day have higher incidence of dental caries.

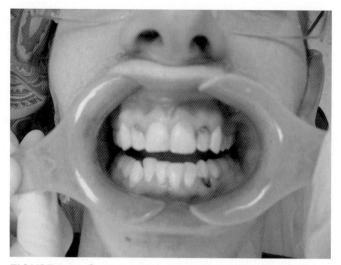

FIGURE 9-7   Dental caries due to frequent carbohydrate consumption.

Knowing about all of the good benefits of saliva confirms that the less saliva, the higher probability of dental caries. A patient with **salivary gland hypofunction** will have a very dry mouth (xerostomia). A sure tip-off is when gloves stick to oral tissues that have a dull appearance. The elderly are at high caries risk due to xerostomia for two main reasons: as we age, we lose the sense of thirst, and many elderly patients will report taking several medications, most of which manifest xerostomia. A dry mouth is one without the benefits of saliva, which has many tooth-protective qualities. When xerostomia is combined with gingival recession there is very high risk for dentinal root caries.

Other groups at risk for dental caries are as follows:

- Anyone with past caries experience: visible caries, restorations placed within the last 3 years
- Those reporting long-term or frequent use of antihypertensive, antidepressant, antihistamine, diuretic, analgesic, and other tranquilizing drugs that decrease saliva
- Patients with diseases that contribute to dry mouth, including cancer, diabetes, anemia, salivary gland dystrophy, stroke, Alzheimer's, Sjögren's syndrome, autoimmune diseases, Parkinson's, and palsy
- Nutrition supplements, such as ma huang and ephedra, that cause dry mouth

- People on a soft diet who do not benefit from crunchy foods bringing good saliva into the oral cavity
- Anyone who reports eating a high-carbohydrate diet and patients who report eating frequent snacks consisting of added sugar: nibblers, grazers, or sippers of sodas and sugared coffee and tea
- People living in an area with a nonfluoridated water supply
- Patients with visible heavy plaque and those with physical limitations that prevent thorough oral hygiene
- Young patients whose parents or caregivers have caries activity[12]

Food for Thought 9-4 identifies groups at risk for dental caries.

DETRIMENTAL EFFECTS OF SODA

The photograph in Figure 9-8 was taken of an adult who reported sipping on two to three sodas per day.

One 12-oz. can of regular soda contains 10 teaspoons of sugar, give or take a few depending on the brand. According to the Academy of General Dentistry website, noncola drinks and canned iced teas are actually more harmful to enamel than Coke, Dr. Pepper, and Pepsi because flavor additives like malic and tartatic and other acids aggressively demineralize enamel. Sprite, Mountain Dew, Ginger-Ale, and Arizona Iced Tea proved to be most harmful, and root beer, brewed

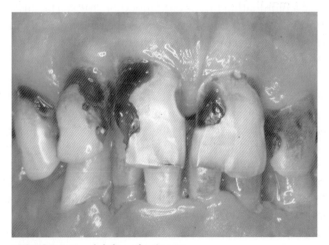

FIGURE 9-8   Adult soda sipper.

black tea, black coffee, and water were the least harmful to enamel.[13] A soda consumed with meals does less damage to teeth than when consumed alone or sipped throughout the day. If your patient wants to drink sodas, suggest drinking the whole can or bottle with a meal. Drinking the soda through a straw may also help reduce enamel demineralization.

Many patients report switching to diet soda to reduce the detrimental effects of regular sugared soda. They should be made aware that diet sodas have citric and **phosphoric acid** with a pH of 2.3 to 2.6 added as flavor enhancers, which erode enamel and very rapidly drops the oral pH to a critical level.

Suggestions for reducing the caries potential of soda in the diet (from the Academy of General Dentistry website) include the following:

- Rinse the mouth with water after drinking soda to eliminate excess sugar that could be used by bacteria to make acid.
- Bypass the teeth by drinking soda from a straw.
- Drink soda from a can rather than a bottle, which can be capped and sipped throughout the day.

COUNSELING PATIENTS

It is important to explain the relationship of food to disease in the oral cavity, and discuss factors that can lessen the impact of sugar in the diet. It is impractical to think that your patients will eliminate all carbohydrates from their diet and unwise to suggest eliminating any favorite food or drink. The best advice would be to rearrange the sequence of foods and beverages within meals and throughout the day. Work at raising the oral pH by including the following cariostatic foods in the diet:

- Cheese (counsel that the protective factors of cheese are lost if eaten with a cookie or cracker or followed with acidic beverage)
  - Aged cheddar
  - Swiss
  - Blue
  - Monterey jack
  - Mozzarella
  - Brie
  - Gouda
- Peanuts

- Artificial sweeteners
- Crunchy foods
- Sugar-free chewing gum

Other good suggestions are as follows:

- If at all possible, reduce frequency of consuming sugary and acidic foods.[14,15]
- Eliminate snacking on carbohydrates before bedtime.
- Combine foods—eat sweets after proteins and fats or follow sugared foods with cheese.
- Combine raw, crunchy foods that stimulate saliva with cooked foods.
- Citrus fruits (citric acid) stimulate saliva production.
- Limit sweetened beverages to meals.[16]
- Eat cookies with milk for benefits of calcium and phosphate.
- Drink iced tea instead of soda—tea will still work as a stimulant but also contains fluoride.[17]
- Drink orange juice with calcium to counteract the acid.[18]
- Do not rush to brush after acidic beverages—let the oral cavity remineralize enamel on its own for about 30 minutes. (Brushing may remove demineralized structure before it has a chance to remineralize.)
- Chewing sugar-free gum stimulates salivary flow that may be effective in neutralizing interproximal plaque acid through mechanical action.
- After sugared gum has lost its flavor, the chewing action can do the same thing as the sugar-free gum.
- Use a fluoridated toothpaste.[19]

Putting This Into Practice

Your client is a 23-year-old female graduate student who presents at your dental practice after a 5-year absence from professional dental care. She reports good health with use of antihistamines as needed for seasonal allergies. Radiographic and clinical examinations reveal five new posterior interproximal carious lesions, and recurrent caries around two existing anterior restorations. A quick inquiry into her diet indicates high intake of carbohydrates, preference for soft foods, and frequent use of sugared

(continued)

breath mints. Home care consists of daily brushing for about 45 seconds and flossing two or three times per week.

1. List all factors in the above scenario that could contribute to dental caries formation, explaining in detail their relationship.
2. Write the advice you would give this client to help reduce future caries development.

WEB RESOURCES

Academy of General Dentistry—Protecting Your Teeth from Food
http://www.agd.org/consumer/topics/childrensnutrition/foodcavities.html

Academy of General Dentistry—Schools Long-Term Soda Deals Kick Kids in the Teeth
http://www.agd.org/consumer/topics/childrensnutrition/soda.html

Academy of General Dentistry—Soda Attack: Soft Drinks, Especially Non-Colas and Iced Tea, Hurt Hard Enamel http://www.agd.org/media/2004/june/drinks.html

National Institute of Nutrition—The Effect of Diet on Dental Health
http://www.nin.ca/public.html/Publications/NinReview/winter97.html#Decay Process

World Sugar Research Organization Information—Sugar and Dental Caries
http://www.wsro.org/public/sugarandhealth/sugaranddentalcaries.html

Wrigley—Sugarfree Chewing Gum and Dental Caries Prevention
http://www.wrigley.com/wrigley/products/dentalprofessionals.asp

REFERENCES

1. Steffen JM. The effects of soft drinks on etched and sealed enamel. *Angle Orthod* 1996;66(6):449–456.
2. Makinen KK, Isotupa KP, Kivilompolo T, et al. Comparison of erythritol and xylitol saliva stimulants in the control of dental plaque and mutans streptococci. *Caries Res* 2001;35(2):129–35.
3. Moss S. Relationship between fluoride, saliva, and diet. *Dent Hyg* 1994;7(4):3–6.
4. Campus G, Lallai MR, Carboni R. Fluoride concentration in saliva after use of oral hygiene products. *Caries Res* 2003;37(1):66–70.
5. Alty CT. The wonders of spit. *RDH* 2003;23(6):54–58.
6. Marshall TA, Levy SM, Broffitt B, et al. Dental caries and beverage consumption in young children. *Pediatrics* 2003;112(3 Pt 1):e184–e191.

7. Effects of sugar on oral health: review and recommendations. *Dent Abstracts* 2002;47:I4.

8. Gilbert D. *The University Record, News and Information Services*. March 29, 1993.

9. Beiswanger BB, Boneta AE, Mau MS, et al. The effect of chewing sugar-free gum after meals on clinical caries incidence. *J Am Dent Assoc* 1998;129(11):1623–1626.

10. Schardt D. Sweet nothings, not all sweeteners are equal. *Nutr Action Healthletter* 2004: 8–11.

11. Featherstone JD. The caries balance: contributing factors and early detection. *J Calif Dent Assoc* 2003;31(2):129–133.

12. Featherstone J. Tipping the scales toward caries control. *Dim Dent Hyg* 2004:20–27.

13. von Fraunhofer JA. Dissolution of dental enamel in soft drinks. *J Gen Dent* 2004;52: 308–312. Available at: http://www.agd.org/library/issue.index.html. Accessed 2007.

14. Loveren C, Duggal MS. Experts' opinions on the role of diet in caries prevention. *Caries Res* 2004;38(Suppl 1):16–23.

15. Levy SM, Warren JJ, Broffitt B, et al. Fluoride, beverages and dental caries in the primary dentition. *Caries Res* 2003;37(3):157–165.

16. Mobley CC. Nutrition and dental caries. *Dent Clin North Am* 2003;47(2):319–336.

17. Behrendt A, Oberste V, Wetzel WE. Fluoride concentration and pH of iced tea products. *Caries Res* 2002;36(6):405–410.

18. Davis R, Marshall T, Qian F, et al. In vitro protection against dental erosion afforded by commercially available, calcium-fortified 100 percent juices. *J Am Dent Assoc* 2007;138:1593–1598.

19. Watt RG, McClone P. Prevention part 2: dietary advice in the dental surgery. *Br Dent J* 2003;195(1):27–31.

SUGGESTED READING

American Academy of Pediatric Dentistry. *Policy paper on early childhood caries (ECC): unique challenges and treatment options*. 2003.

Alvarez JO. Nutrition, tooth development, and dental caries. *Am J Clin Res* 1995;61:410 S–416 S.

Bibby BG, Mundorff SA, Zero DT, et al. Oral food clearance and the pH of plaque and saliva. *J Am Dent Assoc* 1986;112(3):333–337.

Catt D, Fontana M. Is it plaque or biofilm? *J Public Health* 2006: 13–15.

Code of Federal Regulations, Title 21, Vol. 2. US Government Printing Office, April 2002.

Commonwealth Dental Association. *Position paper on diet, nutrition, and the prevention of dental caries and erosion*. http://www.cdauk.com. 2002.

Curnow MM, Pine CM, Burnside G, et al. A randomised controlled trial of the efficacy of supervised toothbrushing in high-caries-risk children. *Caries Res* 2002;36(4): 294–300.

Cury JA, Rebello MA, Del Bel Cury AA. In situ relationship between sucrose exposure and the composition of dental plaque. *Caries Res* 1997;31(5):356–360.

Dong YM, Pearce EI, Yue L, et al. Plaque pH and associated parameters in relation to caries. *Caries Res* 1999;33(6):428–436.

Duggal MS, van Loveren C. Dental considerations for dietary counseling. *Int Dent J* 2001;51(Suppl 1):408–412.

Grein H, Borus J, Tillis T. Combatting America's soda pop obsession. *J Public Health* 2006: 26–28.

Gutkowski S. Chew gum, build enamel. *RDH* 2002:37–38.

Hackett AF, Rugg-Gunn AJ, Murray JJ, et al. Can breast feeding cause dental caries? *Hum Nut Appl nutr* 1984;38(1):23–28.

Harris NO, Garcia-Godoy F. *Primary preventive dentistry*. Upper Saddle River: Prentice Hall; 2003.

Heller KE, Burt BA, Eklund SA. Sugared soda consumption and dental caries in the United States. *J Dent Res* 2001;80(10):1949–1953.

Hornick B. Diet and nutrition implications for oral health. *J Dent Hyg* 2002;76(1):67–78.

Kashket S, DePaola DP. Cheese consumption and the development and progression of dental caries. *J Int Assoc Dent Child* 1990;20(1):3–7.

Krasse B. The Vipeholm dental caries Study: recollections and reflections 50 years later. *J Dent Res* 2001;80(9):1785–1788.

Larsen MJ, Nuvad B. Enamel erosion by some soft drinks and orange juices relative to their pH, buffering effect and contents of calcium phosphate. *Caries Res* 1999;33(1):81–87.

Linke HA, Moss SJ, Arav L, et al. Intra-oral lactic acid production during clearance of different foods containing various carbohydrates. *Z Ernahungswiss* 1997;36(2):191–197.

Linke HA, Riba HK. Oral clearance and acid production of dairy products during interaction with sweet foods. *Ann Nutr Metab* 2001;45(5):202–208.

Luke GA, Gough H, Beeley JA, et al. Human salivary sugar clearance after sugar rinses and intake of foodstuffs. *Caries Res* 1999;33(2):123–129.

Moynihan PJ. Dietary advice in dental practice. *Br Dent J* 2002;193(10):563–568.

Nobre dos Santos M, Melo dos Santos L, Francisco SB, et al. Relationship among dental plaque composition, daily sugar exposure and caries in the primary dentition. *Caries Res* 2002;36(5):347–352.

O'Sullivan EA, Curzon, MEJ. A comparison of acidic dietary factors in children with and without dental erosion. *J Dent Child* 2000;67:186–192.

Pearce EI, Sissons CH, Coleman M, et al. The effect of sucrose application frequency and basal nutrient conditions on the calcium and phosphate content of experimental dental plaque. *Caries Res* 2002;36(2):87–92.

Peressini S. Pacifier use and early childhood caries: an evidence-based study of the literature. *J Can Dent Assoc* 2003;69(1):16–19.

Shannon IL, McCartney JC. Presweetened dry breakfast cereals: potential for dental danger. *ASDC J Dent Child* 1981;48(3):215–218.

Sheiham A. Changing trends in dental caries. *Int J Epidemiol* 1984;13(2):142–147.

Sheiham A. Dietary effects on dental disease. *Public Health Nutr* 2001;4(2B):569–591.

Tinanoff N, Palmer CA. Dietary determinants of dental caries and dietary recommendations for preschool children. *J Public Health Dent* 2000;60(3):197–206.

Touger-Decker R, van Loveren C. Sugars and dental caries. *J Am Clinl Nutr* 2003;78(4): 881 S–892 S.

Woodward M, Walker AR. Sugar consumption and dental caries: evidence from 90 countries. *Br Dent J* 1994;176(8):297–302.

CHAPTER 10

DIET, NUTRITION, AND PERIODONTAL DISEASE

OBJECTIVES

Upon completion of this chapter, the reader will be able to:

1 Identify specific nutrients that assist with building healthy periodontal tissues

2 List nutrients that keep our immune system healthy

3 Outline the immune response when bacteria penetrate the sulcular epithelium and explain the importance of maintaining a healthy sulcular lining

4 Explain the benefit of ample saliva and its relationship to periodontal disease

5 Establish the relationship between a diet of soft retentive foods and periodontal disease

6 Describe how chewing crunchy foods can keep periodontal ligaments and alveolar bone healthy

7 Suggest healthy food choices for patients with periodontal disease

KEY TERMS

Alveolar Bone	Collagen	Detergent Foods
B Complex	Crunchy Foods	Gingivitis
Calcium	Density of Bone	Immune Response

Immune System	Periodontal Ligaments	Soft Foods
Magnesium	Plaque Biofilm	Vitamin A
Periodontal Disease	Saliva	Vitamin D

The connection of what we eat to the occurrence of dental caries is well established: bacteria + carbohydrate = acid that will demineralize enamel. However, the relationship between diet and periodontal disease is not quite as simple and direct. Caries research includes the famous Vipeholm study that clearly established how consumption of simple carbohydrates causes dental decay. But there has been no definitive study linking diet or a specific nutrient to the occurrence or incidence of periodontal disease. Searching for a causative effect between diet and periodontal disease requires control of many variables: poverty ratio, level of attained education, ethnicity, calcium intake, bone density, diabetes, dental visits, smoking, coping mechanisms, genetic response to infection and inflammation, and so on. One can only imagine how difficult it would be to find perfect subjects for a study.

The firm dogma that poor nutrition does not *"cause"* periodontal disease is gradually being eroded as each new piece of research reveals specific nutrient roles in maintaining periodontal health. Research indicates that absence of any one of the following—vitamins A, C, and D; calcium; protein; or complex carbohydrates—in the diet can make the difference between a healthy immune response and continued disease progression.[2-5] More studies are needed to determine if the results can be replicated in different patient groups, and before a statement of a direct link can be made between diet deficiencies and periodontal disease.

There has also been some interest in looking at the relationship between periodontal disease and nutrition in reverse: Instead of questioning whether diet causes/affects periodontal health, researchers are asking if having periodontal disease can affect nutrient intake. Poor periodontal health with its associated bone loss, loose teeth, and swollen bleeding gingiva can cause a desire to choose foods that are easy to chew and will not cause pain.[1]

SPECIFIC NUTRIENTS AND PERIODONTAL HEALTH

Knowing which nutrients keep the tissues healthy and which nutrients can repair diseased tissue will help us counsel patients with active periodontal disease and those at risk, fostering better oral health. **Periodontal disease** is an infection of the periodontium initiated by bacteria within plaque biofilm. A host with a healthy immune system will maintain healthy periodontal tissues, while a host with a poor immune response to bacteria will develop periodontal disease. If the

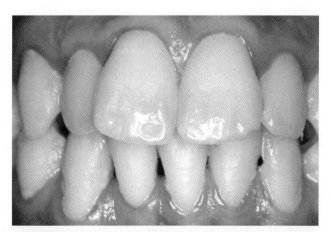

FIGURE 10-1 **Slight plaque-induced gingivitis. Note the very early erythema (redness) of gingival margin.** (Reprinted with permission from Nield-Gehrig J, Willmann D. *Foundations of periodontics for the dental hygienist*, 2nd ed. Baltimore: Lippincott Williams & Wilkins, 2008.)

[handwritten: Periodontitis = connective tissues (ligaments, bone, cementum)]

infection and inflammation are limited to gingival tissues, it is called **gingivitis**. If it extends to connective tissues (periodontal ligaments, bone, and cementum), it is called "periodontitis." Once the bone has been affected, the damage created is irreversible. Figures 10-1 through 10-4 are examples of various degrees of periodontal disease.

Our **immune system** is a complicated yet intelligent process. When bacteria begin their attack on periodontal tissues, the body sends an arsenal of defense organisms to limit their detrimental effects and to repair the damage. This is called an **immune response**. Leukocytes and plasma proteins, delivered through the bloodstream, invade the site of injury, causing swelling and edema. If the host is well nourished and has a healthy immune system, the response mechanism will more than likely take care of the injury and the area will heal. If the host is not well nourished, and the immune system is compromised, it can cause an overzealous attempt to eliminate the bacteria. The body will send an overabundance of immune cells to the area which produce cytokines, along with other enzymes that destroy periodontal fibers and stimulate osteoclastic activity. A well-nourished host with a diet that supplies specific nutrients can be protected against the bacterial assault. Certain nutrients have more influence than others in building, maintaining, and repairing periodontal tissues, some with a single function and others with multiple benefits. Food for Thought 10-1 lists nutrients that assist with tissue synthesis.

[handwritten: Leukocytes + plasma proteins invade site of injury, causing swelling + edema.]

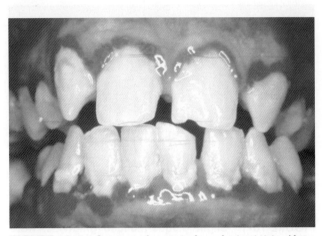

FIGURE 10-2   Severe plaque-induced gingivitis. Note the obvious erythema and edema of the gingival margins and papillae. (Reprinted with permission from Nield-Gehrig J, Willmann D. *Foundations of periodontics for the dental hygienist*, 2nd ed. Baltimore: Lippincott Williams & Wilkins, 2008.)

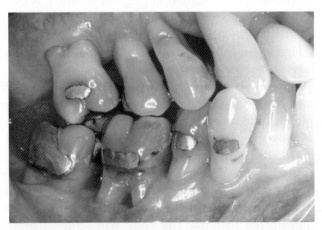

FIGURE 10-3   Aggressive periodontitis in a patient with good plaque control. In aggressive periodontitis, the disease severity typically seems exaggerated given the amount of bacterial plaque. (Reprinted with permission from Nield-Gehrig J, Willmann D. *Foundations of periodontics for the dental hygienist*, 2nd ed. Baltimore: Lippincott Williams & Wilkins, 2008.)

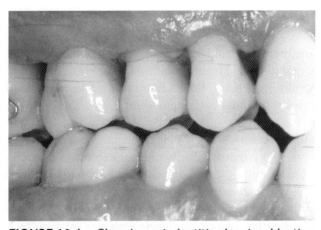

FIGURE 10-4 **Chronic periodontitis showing blunting of the interdental papillae and gingival recession.** (Reprinted with permission from Nield-Gehrig J, Willmann D. *Foundations of periodontics for the dental hygienist*, 2nd ed. Baltimore: Lippincott Williams & Wilkins, 2008.)

🍎 **FOOD FOR THOUGHT 10-1**

NUTRIENTS THAT ASSIST WITH TISSUE SYNTHESIS

- Vitamin A
- B Complex *riboflavin, niacin*
- Vitamin D *dairy magnisium enhances absorbtion of Ca+ Ma builds skelodal bones*
- Calcium *builds skelatal bones*
- Magnesium *build skelatal bones*
- Protein

All of the nutrients together will do the following:

- Build healthy soft and hard periodontal tissues
- Enhance the immune system to fight infection
- Regulate the immune response
- Help with wound healing

BUILDING HEALTHY PERIODONTAL TISSUES

Building and maintaining healthy oral tissue is the body's first line of defense against periodontal disease. Healthy oral tissues are less susceptible to infection and will not require the host to tax its immune system. Once the inflammatory process begins, a strong immune system will be successful in fighting off initial bacterial invasion.

Plaque biofilm develops along the gingival margin where the acquired pellicle has laid down its sticky matrix. As it continues to build its colonies, the mass will spread coronally and apically, drawing the plaque subgingivally to live in the sulcus. Keeping tissue healthy in the sulcus is vital to preventing periodontal disease. The epithelial lining of the gingival sulcus requires an adequate supply of nutrients because it has one of the fastest turnover rates in the body (3 days). Vitamins A, B complex, and D and calcium and magnesium all work to build and maintain healthy soft tissue and bone.

Vitamin A assists in the formation of healthy epithelium and is vital for functioning of the immune system. If a periodontally involved patient has unhealthy pocket lining, it is usually inadvertently curettaged during deposit removal. Eating foods rich in vitamin A will assist the body in forming new healthy epithelial tissue within the sulcus. Without sufficient amounts of vitamin A, there can be an altered response to infection and the scaling site could take longer to heal.

A diet rich in **B complex** vitamins prevents periodontal disease by keeping the immune system healthy and functioning properly. Also, B complex vitamins—thiamin, riboflavin, niacin, pyroxidine, cobalamin, folic acid, biotin, and pantothenic acid—are important in helping form new tissue cells which are needed during the repair process. Because the B complex vitamins are cofactors and work together, a deficiency will involve more than one. Complex carbohydrates such as whole grain breads, brown rice, and pasta are rich in B complex vitamins. In a study conducted on American males, it was determined that increasing whole grains in the diet can reduce the risk of periodontitis.[6]

🍎 FOOD FOR THOUGHT 10-2

Recent research concluded that low serum folate levels in adults can be an indicator of periodontal disease and may be a possible clinical marker for intervention.[8]

Alveolar bone gives support to the roots of our teeth and serves as an anchor for periodontal ligaments so it is necessary for the alveolar process to be well mineralized. We depend on the strength and hardness of the bone to support the function of biting and grinding our food. The presence of certain nutrients during osteoblastic activity will assure development of strong and healthy bone and set the stage for long-term function. Calcified tissues in the body continue to remodel throughout life, so a steady amount of these nutrients is necessary. **Calcium** and **magnesium** are principal minerals that build skeletal bones and teeth. **Vitamin D** enhances the absorption of these two minerals, assisting with bone development and regeneration. During the destructive process of the periodontal disease, bone is resorbed and teeth become loose. Dairy products are a great source of calcium, magnesium, and are fortified with vitamin D. They also contain lactic acid, which has a beneficial effect on periodontal disease.[7] Research shows that decreased dietary intake of calcium results in more severe periodontal disease.[2]

REPAIRING PERIODONTAL INFECTION

Periodontal infection is a wound, and as the body begins the healing/repairing process, good nutrition will greatly assist the conversion of periodontal tissues from a state of disease to one of health. If a diet is lacking in nutrients it can compromise the integrity of the epithelial attachment, making it more permeable to invading bacteria and its resulting infection. Food for Thought 10-3 lists the nutrients that repair diseased or wounded tissue.

🍎 **FOOD FOR THOUGHT 10-3**

NUTRIENTS THAT REPAIR
- Protein
- Vitamin C
- Iron
- Zinc
- Copper
- Selenium

Trace minerals are needed for protein synthesis, which supports growth and maintenance of healthy cells and assists with resistance of infection (see Chapter 3) A well-balanced diet that includes adequate amounts of protein has ample opportunity to make antibodies that target and destroy foreign invaders, whether bacterium, virus, or other toxin.

Including foods rich in vitamin C in the daily diet is important to maintaining healthy periodontium, as it aids in the formation of **collagen**, a cementing substance that assists with wound healing and resisting infection. It also promotes capillary integrity by keeping tissues well nourished at the micro level. Because leukocytes are delivered to the site of bacterial assault through bloodstream, having healthy capillaries is part of a well-functioning immune system. Research has proved that individuals with an inadequate daily intake of vitamin C have a higher incidence of periodontal disease.[3,4] The dietary deficiency disease of vitamin C is scurvy and mimics a really bad case of periodontal disease: gingival tissues appear purplish-red, swollen, and bleed profusely. There is a good

TABLE 10-1   Functions of Nutrients and Minerals

Nutrient	Function	Mineral	Function
Vitamin A	Builds and maintains healthy epithelium Aids immune system	Calcium	Builds and maintains strong alveolar process
B Complex	Forms new cells Keeps immune system healthy	Iron	Forms collagen Aids with wound healing Regulates inflammatory response
Vitamin D	Aids with calcium absorption	Zinc	Forms collagen Aids with wound healing Regulates inflammatory response
Vitamin C	Aids with wound healing Helps the body resist infection	Copper Selenium	Aids with wound healing Prevents harm to cells
Protein	Promotes growth, maintenance, and repair of all body tissues	Magnesium	Works with vitamin D and calcium to build and maintain strong alveolar bone

collagen - a cementing substance that assists w/wound healing + resist infection.

assortment of foods rich in vitamin C such as kiwis; anything with citric acid such as grapefruit, oranges, lemons, and limes; cantaloupe; strawberries; broccoli; and cabbage. All would be great recommendations for patients with periodontal concerns. Vitamin C is also an antioxidant, and along with vitamins A, E, and selenium, will prevent harm to cells and tissues.

Iron, zinc, and copper assist with collagen formation which is necessary during wound healing. They also perform the major function of regulating the inflammatory response which goes haywire in certain individuals, causing more tissue destruction than repair. Table 10-1 identifies all the nutrients and minerals and their function in building, maintaining, and repairing healthy periodontium.

PHYSICAL CONSISTENCY OF FOODS AND THEIR RELATIONSHIP TO PERIODONTAL HEALTH

Whether an individual chooses to include raw **crunchy foods** or mainly soft retentive foods in the diet can impact the health of the periodontium. Crunchy fibrous foods have a beneficial effect on periodontal tissues because the act of chewing will increase salivary flow, which in turn clears foods from the oral cavity. See Table 10-2 for examples of crunchy foods. The longer the food hangs around the oral cavity, the more opportunity for bacteria to feed on carbohydrates and excrete acid. Acid causes demineralization and caries which offer a nidus for plaque bacteria. When bacteria penetrate connective tissue, periodontal disease results. **Saliva** also has antibacterial proteins which protect against periodontal

TABLE 10-2 Crunchy Foods
Raw vegetables: carrots, celery, radishes, broccoli, cauliflower, green beans
Raw fruits: apples, pears
Wasabi peas
Roasted almonds, walnuts, peanuts
Salads
Cole slaw
Water chestnuts
Popcorn

disease.[5] Chewing stimulates saliva production but **soft foods** do not require as much chewing as crunchy foods. Soft, sticky foods are retained longer in a drier mouth, thus creating an opportunity to accumulate more bacteria. The more bacteria in the oral cavity, the more opportunity for infection and inflammation and exaggerated host response.

The act of chewing crunchy foods also produces local exercise for periodontal ligaments and can increase the **density of bone** surrounding the roots of teeth. The more exercise **periodontal ligaments** get, the stronger their attachment is. The denser the alveolar bone, the stronger the support for the teeth. The healthier and stronger the periodontal structures, the less restricted the diet is, making the body better nourished and healthier overall.[1]

Food for Thought 10-4 lists benefits to the periodontium from eating chewy and crunchy foods. Food for Thought 10-5 lists the benefits of good nutrition on periodontal disease.

🍎 FOOD FOR THOUGHT 10-4

BENEFITS OF CHEWY AND CRUNCHY FOODS IN THE DIET

- Stimulate saliva production
- Exercise periodontal ligaments
- Increase bone density surrounding the tooth

🍎 FOOD FOR THOUGHT 10-5

BENEFITS OF GOOD NUTRITION ON PERIODONTAL DISEASE

- Helps tissues resist infection
- Strengthens and maintains the epithelial barrier
- Promotes the repair of damaged tissues

🍎 FOOD FOR THOUGHT 10-6

Years ago, it was thought that chewing fibrous foods could remove plaque at the gingival margin, but that theory has been proved incorrect. There is no such thing as **"detergent" foods**, and the act of chewing fibrous foods will not increase gingival keratinization.

COUNSELING PATIENTS

It is a known fact that disease, oral medications, and unhealthy lifestyle choices can increase a person's risk for periodontal disease. Your patient cannot change the fact that he or she has a disease or is taking a medication, but he or she does have free choice to change the eating habits. It is the dental clinician's responsibility to counsel periodontally involved patients to make wise food choices that will enhance oral health, thereby improving total overall health. Your goal in counseling periodontally involved patients should be to initiate awareness of how periodontal health relies on a balance between bacterial factors and the host environment. The dental clinician can influence the overall quality of a diet and encourage good nutrition for general and oral health by making suggestions to modify food choices. See Table 10-3. Nutritional recommendations for periodontal health are the same as those suggested for overall health including:

- Follow the U.S. Department of Agriculture MyPyramid
- Include foods rich in calcium, B complex vitamins, protein, complex carbohydrates, and antioxidants
- Follow the Dietary Guidelines for Healthy Americans

TABLE 10-3	Food Sources of Nutrients
Nutrient	**Foods Source**
Vitamin A	Carrots, sweet potatoes, pumpkin, spinach, collards, kale, green beans, red peppers
B Complex	Fortified cereals, pork, liver, brewer's yeast, soybeans, peas, nuts, fortified whole grains, dairy products
Vitamin C	Guava, red and green peppers, kiwi, citrus fruit, canteloupe, strawberries, broccoli, cabbage, Brussel sprouts
Protein	Beef, pork, eggs, milk, fish, poultry, legumes, tofu and soy products
Complex carbohydrate	Whole grain bread, rice, pasta, oat meal, all bran cereal, corn, yams, peas, lentils
Calcium	Milk, cheese, yogurt, fortified orange juice, tofu, tahini, sardines, turnip greens, okra, kale
Vitamin D	Milk, soy beverage, trout, salmon, sardines, tuna

[Handwritten annotations: "Aids immune system / epithelium"; "immune system / forms new cells"; "healing wounds / ↓infection"; "↑grow"; "↑ + maintains alveolar process"; "aids in calcium absorbtion"]

- Take a daily dose of the recommended daily allowance (RDA) for vitamins and minerals
- Include crunchy, chewy foods in the diet to bring healthy saliva into the oral cavity

Putting This Into Practice

Your patient is a 29-year-old single male with a history of infrequent dental visits. Results of initial assessment:

Medical/Dental

- Weight 185 lb, height 5 ft 10 in.
- Blood pressure 140/90 mm Hg
- No significant disease factors

Intra-/Extraoral Examination

- Multiple facial piercings—bilateral ear lobe, left nares of nose, corner of right eyebrow, and tongue
- Clicking of temporomandibular joint (TMJ) upon opening
- Bilateral swollen submandibular lymph nodes
- Coated tongue
- Bilateral linea-alba

Periodontal/Gingival Examination

- Generalized marginal and papillary redness
- Heavy marginal plaque and light subgingival calculus
- Localized blunted papilla in mandibular anterior/facial and lingual
- Moderate generalized bleeding upon probing
- Pocket depth range 3 to 6 mm
- No significant recession or furcal involvement

Dental Charting

- Class I amalgam restorations in first molars
- Porcelain crown no. 9

(continued)

- Suspicious area occlusal no. 31
- Impacted third molars

Nutritional Survey Assessment

- Irregular eating habits
- Patient is a musician and is primarily nocturnal
- Meals consist of fast food and convenient microwavable meals
- Lactose intolerant
- Avoids foods with crunchy consistency due to popping in TMJ

1. Based on the assessment information, evaluate the need for nutritional counseling and explain where your time could best be spent.
2. Outline the source of his nutrient deficiency based on the information given regarding his eating habits.
3. List some ideal foods with specific nutrients and state why the food/nutrient is needed in his diet.
4. Based on your suggestions, what do you expect in the way of improvement of periodontal health?

WEB RESOURCES

American Academy of Periodontology www.perio.org.

UCLA Periodontics Information Center http://www.dent.ucla.edu/pic/links.html.

REFERENCES

1. Raymer RE, Sheiham A. Numbers of natural teeth, diet, and nutritional status in US adults. *J Dent Res* 2007;86(12):1171–1175.
2. Nishida M, Grossi SG, Dunford RG, et al. Calcium and the risk for periodontal disease. *J Periodontol* 2000;71(7):1057–1066.
3. Lowe G, Woodward M, Rumley A, et al. Total tooth loss and prevalent cardiovascular disease in men and women: possible roles of citrus fruit consumption, vitamin C, and inflammatory and thrombotic variables. *J Clin Epidemiol* 2003;56(7):694–700.
4. Chapple H, Milward MR, Dietrich T. The prevalence of inflammatory periodontitis is negatively associated with serum antioxidant concentrations. *Int J Clin Pract* 2007;61(10):1705–1707.

A, Arataki T, et al. Relationship between antimicrobial protein
d periodontitis. *J Periodontol* 2008;79(2):310–322.

v, Franz M, et al. Whole grain and fiber intakes and periodontitis
.in Nut 2006;83(6):1395–1400.

urota T, Uchida K, et al. Intake of dairy products and periodontal disease:
.ia Study. *J Periodontol* 2008;79(1):131–137.

, Kuo HK, Lai YL. The association between serum folate levels and periodontal
case in older adults: data from the National Health and Nutrition Examination Survey
2001/02. *J Am Geriatric Soc* 2007;55(1):108–113.

FOOD GUIDELINES

PART IV

FOOD GUIDELINES

CHAPTER 11

CHOOSING FOODS WISELY

OBJECTIVES

Upon completion of this chapter, the reader will be able to:

1 Identify protocols individuals can employ that will assure healthy food choices
2 List important healthy eating guidelines that are common throughout the world
3 Choose foods wisely to prevent disease
4 Demonstrate four steps in keeping food safe
5 Discuss common kitchen dangers
6 Explain the U.S. Department of Agriculture's (USDA) MyPyramid and discuss key points in using it as a resource to healthy eating
7 Counsel patients on how to locate guidelines for making healthy food selections and using MyPyramid

KEY TERMS

5-a-day
Cruciferous
Diet
Dietary Guidelines

Energy Balance
Food-Borne Illnesses
Kitchen Dangers

Safe Food Handling
MyPyramid
Unified Dietary Guidelines

When we are feeling well, we wish for many things; bigger houses, nicer car, new fashionable clothes—the list goes on and on. But when we are ill, the only thing we wish for is restored health. Because there is a scientific link between good nutrition and good health, why would not we want to make wise food choices? But how do you know if you are choosing foods wisely to maintain good health and keep you disease-free? The amount of nutrition information is daunting, some of it is credible and some are not completely accurate. How do you filter through the information to choose what is best for your family while enjoying the process of preparing and eating tasty meals? The answer is to follow guidelines developed by credible sources with proven track records that will lead us through life, healthy and disease-free. Most countries have developed plans for good nutrition that include guidelines and pictorial representations of culturally preferred foods as suggestions to help maintain health. Following established dietary guidelines, making our food selections according to a healthy food graphics, and utilizing good food-handling and safety measures ensure a course for better health and possibly a longer life.

DIETARY GUIDELINES

Dietary Guidelines are typically government documents carefully crafted by nutritional experts that, if followed, will serve as a foundation for making good food choices for healthy eating habits to prevent certain chronic diseases. Dietary Guidelines for Americans made its debut in 1980 and is updated, by law, every 5 years (http://www.health.gov/DietaryGuidelines/.) The format has changed dramatically over the years from simple bulleted statements to a lengthy document that includes food selection for age-groups, necessity for physical activity and weight management, and food sources of specific nutrients. The U.S. guidelines were developed by nutritional experts from the U.S. Department of Agriculture (USDA) and Department of Health and Human Services (HHS). Its purpose is to guide Americans, over the age of 2, to choose a healthy, well-balanced diet and to set standards for federal nutrition programs such as school lunch programs.

Other countries have established their own guidelines, taking into account cultural preferences and seasonal availability of foods. Because we live in a globally connected world, many of our patients may be following their home country's nutritional guidelines and for better compliance while counseling, it is wise to make suggestions that align with what they use. Reading other countries' nutritional guidelines emphasizes the fact that the intended use for all is to keep people healthy. The following is a sampling of dietary guidelines from around the world, many with similar messages as the United States, and all with good advice that is helpful wherever you live.

Australia

- Enjoy a wide variety of nutritious foods.
- Eat plenty of vegetables, legumes, and fruits.
- Eat plenty of cereals (including breads, rice, pasta, and noodles), preferably whole grain.
- Include lean meat, fish, poultry, and/or alternatives.
- Include milks, yogurts, cheeses, and/or alternatives. Reduced-fat varieties should be chosen, where possible.
- Drink plenty of water (http://www.nhmrc.gov.au/publications/synopses/dietsyn.htm).

Take care to:

- Limit saturated fat and moderate total fat intake.
- Choose foods low in salt.
- Limit your alcohol intake if you choose to drink.
- Consume only moderate amounts of sugars and foods containing added sugars.
- Prevent weight gain: be physically active and eat according to your energy needs.
- Care for your food: prepare and store it safely.
- Encourage and support breastfeeding.

Canada

- Enjoy various foods.
- Emphasize cereals, breads, other grain products, vegetables, and fruits.
- Choose lower-fat dairy products, leaner meats, and food prepared with little or no fat.
- Achieve and maintain a healthy body weight by enjoying regular physical activity and healthy eating.
- Limit salt, alcohol, and caffeine (http://www.hc-sc.gc.ca/fn-an/food-guide-aliment/index_e.html).

Germany

- Choose from among many different foods.
- Eat cereal products several times per day and plenty of potatoes.
- Eat fruits and vegetables often—take "5-a-day."
- Consume milk and dairy products daily; fish once a week; and meat, sausages, and eggs in moderation.
- Restrict dietary fat to 70 to 90 g/d, preferably of plant origin.

- Use sugar and salt in moderation—be creative in using herbs and spices.
- Drink plenty of liquids—water is vitally necessary. Drink alcohol in moderation.
- Make sure your dishes are prepared gently and taste well.
- Take your time and enjoy eating.
- Watch your weight and stay active (www.iuns.org/adhering-bodies/report/germany.htm).

Great Britain

- Enjoy your food.
- Eat different foods as shown on the Eat Well Plate.
- Eat the right amount to be a healthy weight—energy needs are dependent on gender, age, body size, and activity level.
- Eat plenty of foods rich in starch and fiber.
- Eat plenty of fruits and vegetables.
- Do not eat too many foods that contain a lot of fat.
- Do not have sugary foods and drinks too often.
- Do not eat too many foods high in salt, and cut down on the amount of salt added in cooking and at the table (http://www.nutrition.org.uk/upload/BNF%20Healthy%20Eating(5)(1).pdf).

India

- Overall energy intake should be restricted to levels commensurate to the sedentary occupations of the affluent, so obesity is avoided.
- Highly refined and polished cereals should be avoided in preference to undermilled cereals.
- Green leafy vegetables (a source not only of carotene but also of linolenic acid derivatives) should be included at least in levels recommended by International Conference on Dietary Guidelines.
- Edible fat intake need not exceed 40 g, and total fat intake should be limited to levels at which fat will provide no more than 20% of total energy. The use of clarified butter should be restricted for special occasions and should not be a regular daily feature.
- Intake of sugar and sweets should be restricted.
- High salt intake should be restricted (http://www.ninindia.org/).

Ireland

- Enjoy your food.
- Eat different foods, using the Food Pyramid as a guide.

- Eat the right amount of food to be a healthy weight, and exercise regularly. Foods with a lot of fiber fill you up quickly, so you will be less likely to want high-fat foods. This will help you be a healthy weight.
- Eat four or more portions of fruit and vegetables every day. Try to get into the habit of having at least one portion of fruit juice, fruit, or vegetable at each meal.
- Eat more foods rich in starch—breads and cereals (especially whole grain), potatoes, pasta and rice, and fruit and vegetables.
- Reduce the amount of fatty foods you eat, especially saturated fats. Make lower-fat choices whenever possible. Grill, boil, oven-bake, or stir-fry in very little fat instead of deep frying. Try eating fewer foods from the top of the Food Pyramid.
- If you drink alcohol, keep within sensible limits. Preferably, drink with meals and try to make every second day an alcohol-free day.
- Use various seasonings; try not to always rely on salt to flavor foods. Use herbs, spices, and black pepper as alternatives.
- If you drink or eat snacks containing sugar, limit the number of times you take them throughout the day. This is particularly important for children's growing teeth (http://www.fsai.ie/scientific/nutrition/nutrition.asp).

Korea

- Eat various foods.
- Maintain your ideal body weight.
- Eat sufficient amounts of protein.
- Eat 20% total energy intake from fats.
- Drink milk every day.
- Choose a diet low in salt.
- Maintain your teeth's health.
- Restrict smoking and drinking of alcohol and caffeinated beverages.
- Maintain a balance between energy intake and expenditure.
- Enjoy homemade meals to be happy with families (http://www.afic.org/ National%20Dietary%20Guidelines%20for%20Korea.htm).

Philippines

- Eat various foods every day. (Eat a balanced diet from various foods; pay particular attention to your food needs during pregnancy and lactation; prepare meals for your children that are varied, complete, and adequate for their growth and development; support the elderly with a diet suitable to their conditions; choose ready-to-eat foods with high nutritional value.)

- Promote breastfeeding and proper weaning. (Learn about and promote the advantages and value of breastfeeding; learn the techniques of successful breastfeeding; breastfeed for as long as there is milk; start supplementary foods when the baby is 4- to 6-months-old.)
- Achieve and maintain desirable body weight. (Weigh yourself and the members of your family regularly and behave accordingly; maintain energy balance to desirable body weight; exercise regularly—it is good for you.)
- Eat clean and safe food. (Learn to prevent food-borne diseases; practice safe food storage, handling, preparation, and service.)
- Practice a healthy lifestyle. (Be moderate in what you eat and drink; avoid smoking and control stress; maintain good dental health.)
  (http://www.fnri.dost.gov.ph/index.php?option=content&task=view&id=747)

United States

- Aim for a healthy weight.
- Be physically active each day.
- Let the Food Pyramid guide your food choices.
- Choose various grains daily, especially whole grains.
- Choose various fruits and vegetables daily.
- Keep food safe to eat.
- Choose a diet that is low in saturated fat and cholesterol and moderate in total fat.
- Choose beverages and food to moderate intake of sugars.
- Choose and prepare foods with less salt.
- If you drink alcoholic beverages, do so in moderation (http://www.health.gov/DietaryGuidelines/).

UNIFIED DIETARY GUIDELINES

Before 1999, major health organizations for cancer, heart disease, diabetes, and hypertension each had their own set of dietary guidelines for people to follow to reduce their risk of the specific disease. It is not unusual for a person to have more than one disease, such as the combination of diabetes and heart disease or having hypertension and hypercholesteremia. Having several guidelines to follow is confusing, and oftentimes they fall by the wayside. To help with compliance, the organizations united their suggestions and developed one set of guidelines for healthy eating—the Unified Dietary Guidelines. The **Unified Dietary Guidelines** have been approved by the American Cancer Society, American Heart Association,

American Dietetic Association, American Academy of Pediatrics, and National Institute of Health, and if followed, will reduce the risk for many chronic diseases. The following is a list of their suggestions:

- Eat various foods; choose most of what you eat from plant sources.
- Eat six or more servings of breads, cereals, pasta, and grains each day.
- Choose five or more servings of vegetables per day.
- Eat high-fat foods sparingly, especially those from animal sources. Choose fats and oils with 2 g or less saturated fat per tablespoon, such as liquid and tub margarines, canola oil, and olive oil.
- Keep your intake of simple sugars to a minimum.
- Balance the number of calories you eat with the number you use each day.
- Eat less than 6 g of salt (sodium chloride) per day (2,400 mg of sodium).
- Have no more than one alcoholic drink per day if you are a woman and no more than two if you are a man.

5-A-DAY PROGRAM

Even with the major health organizations recommending the **5-A-Day** program for fruits and vegetables, Americans consume less than three servings a day. Food for Thought 11-1 contains useful information for distinguishing fruits and vegetables. Unless fruit and vegetable dishes are dripping in butter or sugar, they are considered an excellent low-fat source of vitamins, minerals, and fiber. Avocados, coconut, and olives are the exception because they are high in fat, but remember, not all fat is bad. The National Cancer Institute (branch of the National Institutes of Health) refers to fruit and vegetables as the original "fast food." Grapes, cherry tomatoes, and bananas can be eaten on the spot without any preparation.

🍎 FOOD FOR THOUGHT 11-1

DISTINGUISHING FRUITS AND VEGETABLES

Fruits contain seeds.
Vegetables are plants that do not contain seeds.

Any fruit or vegetable "counts" toward the goal of five-a-day, but knowing which are rich in vitamins A and C as well those that are considered **cruciferous** (plant family that has four leaves placed like a cross) will help in choosing a good variety. The National Cancer Institute recommends choosing one fruit or vegetable high in vitamin A and one high in vitamin C per day, and several cruciferous vegetables each week to guard against certain cancers. Food for Thought 11-2 and 11-3 identify cruciferous vegetables and those fruits and vegetables considered good sources of fiber. Table 11-1 indicates source of vitamins A and C in fruits and vegetables.

🍎 **FOOD FOR THOUGHT 11-2**

CRUCIFEROUS VEGETABLES

- Bok choy
- Broccoli
- Brussel sprouts
- Cabbage
- Cauliflower

🍎 **FOOD FOR THOUGHT 11-3**

GOOD SOURCES OF FIBER

- Apples
- Bananas
- Blackberries/blueberries/raspberries/strawberries
- Brussel sprouts
- Carrots
- Cherries
- Cooked beans and peas
- Dates/figs
- Grapefruits/oranges
- Kiwi
- Pears
- Prunes
- Spinach
- Sweet potatoes

Fresh, frozen, canned, or dried fruits and vegetables all provide vitamins, minerals, and fiber; fruit and vegetable juice also provide vitamins and minerals.

TABLE 11-1 Good Source of Vitamin		
	A	**C**
Acorn squash	×	
Apricots	×	×
Bell peppers		×
Broccoli		×
Brussel sprouts		×
Cabbage		×
Cantaloupe	×	×
Carrots	×	
Cauliflower		×
Chili peppers		×
Collards	×	×
Grapefruit		×
Honeydew melon		×
Kale	×	
Kiwi		×
Leaf lettuce	×	
Mangos	×	×
Mustard greens	×	×
Oranges		×
Pineapple		×
Plums		×
Potato with skin		×
Pumpkin	×	
Romaine lettuce	×	

Continued

TABLE 11-1 *(continued)*		
	A	C
Spinach	×	×
Strawberries		×
Sweet potatoes	×	
Tangerines		×
Tomatoes		×
Watermelon		×
Winter squash	×	

A wise shopper, however, knows it makes a difference as to what form of fruit or vegetable is bought:

1. Fresh is best. Food is freshest if picked ripe off the vine and eaten immediately. If picked unripe, it may not have had enough time to accumulate all its nutrients. Many fruits and vegetables are harvested too early and then sprayed to retard spoilage as they travel to the grocery store and sit on the produce shelf waiting for purchase.
2. Frozen is the next best choice after fresh with nutrient levels being high. When choosing produce from the frozen food section, shake the bag to make sure the contents move around. If the contents do not move around and the bag is one big block of ice, this indicates that the contents have been allowed to thaw, which causes the nutrients to leach out of the food and into the water. When refrozen, the nutrients are in the block of ice instead of in the vegetables themselves.
3. Canned is the least desirable, as the canning process requires intense heat, which can destroy many of the B vitamins.

FOOD PYRAMIDS AND GRAPHICS

Illustrated food selection graphics are another dynamic way to visually give patients ideas for making better food choices for overall health. The graphics are geometric and depending on the country, can be triangular, circular, square, or three-dimensional (3D) pyramids with sections that represent various food groups. The idea is that the larger the section, the more foods in that group should

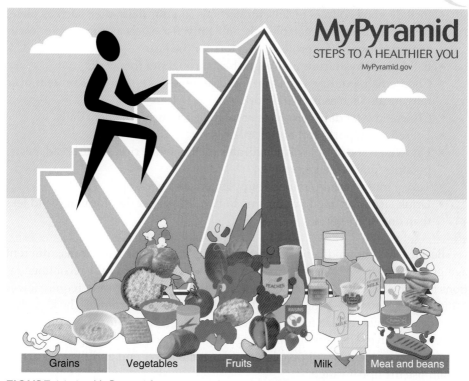

MyPyramid
STEPS TO A HEALTHIER YOU
MyPyramid.gov

| Grains | Vegetables | Fruits | Milk | Meat and beans |

FIGURE 11-1   MyPyramid. (Reprinted from USDA, MyPyramid.gov; accessed June 9, 2008.)

be eaten. A picture is worth a thousand words and having examples of foods in each group can trigger ideas for similar foods that may not be pictured, allowing for greater food choices.

The U.S. pyramid, formerly Food Guide Pyramid, is called **MyPyramid**, and was updated by the USDA and Department of Health and Human Services (Figure 11-1). Medical and nutrition organizations/groups are able to take the concept of MyPyramid and adapt it to make their own recommendations, taking main staples and cultural preferences into considerations. Just as an example, Mayo Clinic website has several colorful pictorial food graphics based on MyPyramid that depict food selections for Asians, mediterraneans, latinos, vegetarians as well as their own design for healthy eating. http://www.mayoclinic.com/health/healthy-diet/NU00190.

Points to consider when interpreting food pyramids are as follows:

- A healthy diet should be combined with exercise and weight control.
- Eat whole grains versus refined at most meals for satiety and more stable blood glucose levels.

- Include good sources of unsaturated fats in your daily diet, such as olive, canola, and other vegetable oils and fatty fish such as salmon, to lower cholesterol and offer protective factors for the heart.
- Eat various fresh fruits and vegetables throughout the week.
- Choose fish, poultry, eggs, nuts, and legumes as a source of protein over fatty meats such as beef and pork.
- Choose low-fat dairy products or take a calcium supplement daily.
- Eat red meat, pork, and butter sparingly.
- Eat refined and simple carbohydrates such as white rice, white bread, pasta, potatoes, and sweets sparingly.
- Take a multivitamin/mineral supplement as a back-up.
- Drink alcohol in moderation: one to two drinks per day for males and less than one drink per day for females.

Because MyPyramid is based on a 2,000-calorie diet for Americans, different age-groups and those with differing activity levels should alter the recommendations to fit their needs. Children have different food preferences and require fewer calories. See Figure 11-2 for the USDA Children's Food Pyramid. Those with a sedentary lifestyle require fewer calories than those who are in a state of growth or are very active. The serving-size suggestions for each food group are given in a range, so inactive or small people should use the lower end and the very active should use the upper range.

BALANCING DIET AND PHYSICAL ACTIVITY

In 1994, the National Weight Control Registry was created to keep track of and identify the habits of individuals who were successful in losing and maintaining weight. More than 5,000 individuals are now in the database, making it one of the largest studies of its kind. Years of research reveal why these individuals were successful in losing an average of 60 lb and maintaining the loss for at least 5 years: they were highly motivated and had increased their daily physical activity level. Weight loss was not necessarily a result of the foods they chose or excluded from their diets. Physical activity and a sensible diet work together for better health.

Energy balance is when calories consumed are adequate for maintenance or growth. When there is an excess of calories consumed—more than needed for maintenance—weight increases. A decrease in calories results in weight loss. Weight gain or loss is referred to as "energy imbalance." We need to eat each day to provide our bodies with energy to keep our hearts beating, lungs expanding, liver and kidneys filtering waste, and sodium pumps maintaining water balance.

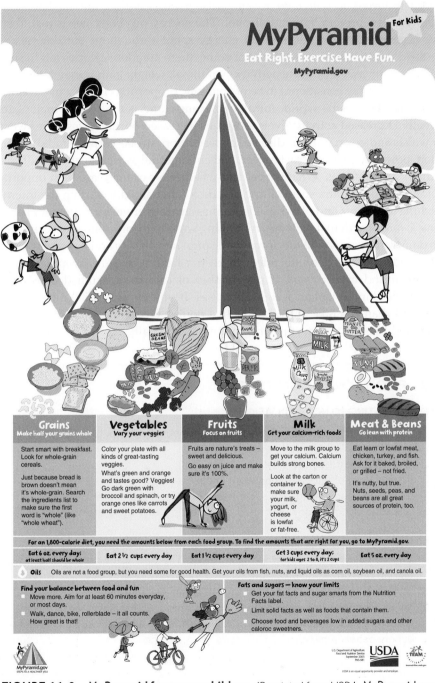

FIGURE 11-2 MyPyramid for young children. (Reprinted from USDA, MyPyramid.gov; accessed June 9, 2008.)

Energy (calories) is delivered to all parts of our bodies from metabolism of carbohydrates, protein, fat, and alcohol. The energy our body needs just to stay alive accounts for two-thirds of all energy spent throughout the day, leaving one-third for our physical activity. For some, there are more calories left to spend than are spent, and if physical activity is minimal, weight gain is inevitable.

Obesity is now considered to be of epidemic proportions not just in the United States, but all over the world, for all age-groups, and is the second major cause of death. Decreased activity levels as well as increased portion sizes have swelled our waists and given us heart disease, hypertension, stroke, certain kinds of cancer (colon, postmenopausal breast cancer, and endometrial as well as others still being studied), and diabetes. What we eat and whether we exercise are both important choices to make. Hours spent sitting at a desk (or chairside), surfing the Internet, watching television, and playing video games create overweight, sedentary people. Being aware of activity levels and rethinking ways to incorporate physical activity into daily routines prevent the downward spiral into obesity and its accompanying diseases. It takes a conscious effort to keep a healthy weight, keeping track of calories in and calories out. If the number of calories consumed consistently exceeds the number spent, weight increases. If you expend 3,500 more calories each week than you take in, you will lose a pound. Over time, that adds up. Food for Thought 11-4 lists some tips on avoiding weight gain.

🍎 FOOD FOR THOUGHT 11-4

TIPS FOR EATING TO NOT GAIN WEIGHT

1. Practice portion control. Eat everything you normally eat, but make a conscious effort to eat a little less.
2. Chew sugarless gum.
3. Enjoy a bowl of unbuttered popcorn in the evening.
4. Give in to your craving with a few bites of the food you desire.
5. Chew slowly and enjoy your food. Avoid eating when you are stressed or feel rushed.
6. Select low-fat dairy products.
7. Choose whole grain vs. refined grain foods. The bulk will give you a sense of fullness quicker.
8. Sip water throughout the day and munch on raw vegetables.
9. Try dividing your daily ratio of food into six small meals versus three large meals. It keeps your metabolism working at top efficiency and you would not feel as hungry between meals.

Continued on next page

10. Avoid using a lot of sauces and gravies.
11. Choose snacks that require some work, like cracking nuts and peeling fruit. The effort in preparation will reduce amount eaten.
12. Eat for better health, not to lose weight, and the pounds will gradually roll off.

The recommended 30 minutes of physical activity per day does not have to be accomplished all at once. Short bursts of activity throughout the day are also acceptable, although sustained activity levels are best for weight loss. If exercise has not been part of your daily routine, remember to start out slow and gradually increase intensity. Starting out fast and furious can only lead to pain and injury. Food for Thought 11-5 offers suggestions on weight loss.

🍎 FOOD FOR THOUGHT 11-5

SUGGESTIONS ON WEIGHT LOSS

Aim for slow weight loss versus rapid weight loss.
Stay away from diets that promise rapid results.
Reducing your *weekly* diet by 3,500 calories will result in a 1 lb weight loss.

All types of physical activity are beneficial. Aerobic exercise speeds up your heart rate and breathing, keeping the circulatory system strong. Strength training, such as lifting weights, helps maintain bone strength and prevent osteoporosis. Stretching while dancing or doing yoga can increase flexibility, making other activities more enjoyable. The following are examples of moderate exercise that can burn 100 to 200 extra calories per day:

- Washing and waxing a car for 45 minutes
- Gardening for 45 minutes
- Raking leaves for 30 minutes
- Walking a 15-minute mile for 30 minutes
- Pushing a baby stroller for 30 minutes
- Shooting baskets for 30 minutes
- Riding a bike for 30 minutes
- Swimming laps for 20 minutes

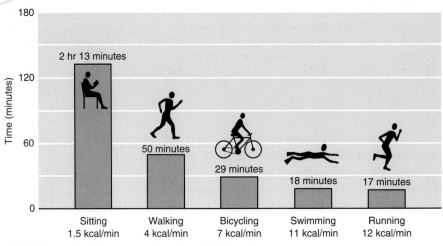

FIGURE 11-3 **Time needed to burn 200 kcal.**

Figure 11-3 details the time needed to burn 200 kcal.

Other suggestions to incorporate physical activity into your day include the following:

- Limit time spent in front of the TV or computer and spend the time moving your body.
- Always opt for the stairs versus elevators or escalators.
- Ride the exercise bike as you watch TV.
- Dance to your favorite music.
- Send children outside to play instead of sitting in front of the TV or computer.
- Trade a sit-down lawnmower for push mower.
- Park as far away from work, mall, or arena entrances as possible, and while doing so, think about how fortunate you are to be healthy enough to walk the distance.
- If safe, let the kids ride their bikes to school or sports practice once a week.
- Form a walking group in your neighborhood and establish a specific meeting time and place.
- Conduct a walking meeting instead of sitting around a conference table.
- Walk with coworkers to restaurants for lunch.

EATING TO DECREASE RISK OF CANCER

A nutrition text would not be complete without including suggestions on what we should and should not eat to decrease the risk of cancer. If approximately one-third of all cancer in the world can be prevented with proper diet and physical activity, it is worth learning to choose which foods are best, and those we should avoid. Decide to make one small dietary change and practice it for 3 weeks and then choose another. Before long you will be incorporating more grains, fruits, and vegetables into meals that will change body fat ratio in just a few months. Just say "no" to high-fat and sugared foods (but maybe not to chocolate).

Incorporating daily activity is suggested to decrease cancer risk. The human body was designed to move, and we should move it until the day of our last sunset. Park farther from the entrance, place frequently used objects so you have to stretch (reach) to get them, or exaggerate movements when doing simple chores like folding clothes. Small changes can lead to big improvements if practiced over time. The American Institute for Cancer Research publication titled Food, Nutrition, Physical Activity and the Prevention of Cancer: A Global Perspective suggests the following:

- Be as lean as possible within your normal body weight range.
- Be physically active as part of everyday life.
- Limit consumption of calorie-dense food (those high in fat and sugar) and avoid sugary drinks.
- Eat mostly foods of plant origin—fruits, vegetables, and whole grains.
- Limit intake of red meat (beef, pork, and lamb) and avoid processed meats, such as bacon, sausage, and lunchmeat—bologna, ham, and salami.
- Limit your intake of alcoholic beverages.
- Limit your salt intake.
- Aim to meet your nutritional needs through diet alone.
- Mothers should breastfeed their babies as it is good for both mother and child; it lowers the risk of breast cancer and the child is less likely to become obese.
- Cancer survivors should be encouraged to follow the report on recommendations for cancer prevention, and of course, seek and take the advice of a trained nutrition professional.

DIETS

Anyone who eats food is on a diet because the literal meaning of the word "diet" is food and drink regularly consumed. But a more common meaning of **diet** is restriction of food and drink, and that is what most people think of when we say we are on a "diet." With obesity being of global concern, many of our patients presenting with oral disease—dental caries or periodontal concerns—will be on a specific diet that must be considered when counseling to prevent/reduce oral disease. Demonstrating respect for a patient's wish to follow a particular diet enforces your concern for their overall health, and earns respect for the suggestions you make for better oral health.

There are many diet or weight reduction organizations that are very specific with food choices and eating suggestions, even to the point of providing exclusive prepackaged food products. The following is a list of some of the more common diets that patients may be following and that should be researched before offering (instead of to include in) suggestions to assure better compliance.

Zone Diet

The Zone Diet was developed by Dr. Barry Sears and published in his best seller book aptly titled The Zone in 1995. Dr. Sears, a well-known research scientist who has spent more than 30 years studying and writing about lipids and hormones and their effect on heart disease, uses the premise that if we treat food as a drug, we can keep ourselves healthy and disease-free (http://www.zonediet.com/). The five simple components to follow with this diet are as follows:

1. Balance every meal and snack with carbohydrate, protein, and fat. Meal composition should be 40-30-30, respectively
2. Include anti-inflammatory Omega 3 fats
3. Include polyphenols (phytochemicals) that are found abundantly in fruits and vegetables for anti-inflammatory and antioxidant benefits
4. Moderately exercise for 30 minutes 6 days a week
5. Take daily supplements

Meals prepared for individuals on this diet are fairly balanced but if counseling a patient subscribing to this diet, it would be important to suggest foods high in Omega 3 and fruits and vegetables high in antioxidants.

Atkins Diet

The Atkins Diet is the most marketed and well-known low-carbohydrate nutritional program. Dr. Robert Atkins found himself in need of a way to lose weight in the 1960s and adapted a diet published in the Journal of American Medical Association to serve his needs. In 1998, after many years of successful weight loss and maintenance, he published the diet in his best selling book titled Dr. Atkins Diet Revolution. The success of the diet depends on the individual's ability to know how much carbohydrate there is in each food choice. Most eating choices are from the protein food group. Visit this link for an example of a low-carbohydrate food pyramid: http://lowcarbdiets.about.com/OD/whattoeat/IG/Low-Carb-FOOD-Pyramid/lowcarbpyramid1-IG.htm. Counseling patients on this diet can be tricky as proportion of food choices are not according to what is usually suggested in MyPyramid. If counseling a patient on this diet, it would be important to suggest food choices illustrated on the low-carbohydrate food pyramid.

South Beach Diet

The South Beach Diet was developed in 1990s by Miami cardiologist Dr. Arthur Agastston and emphasizes eating good carbohydrates and good fats. Foods with a high glycemic index and saturated or trans fats are eliminated. Success of this diet depends on knowing which foods are acceptable versus those that are prohibited. The first phase of the diet lasts 2 weeks and allows only specific foods, called "authorized foods," to eliminate food cravings for sugar and refined starches. If counseling a patient on this diet, it would be important to know which phase of the diet your patient is in and to have a list of foods you can and cannot suggest (http://www.southbeachdiet.com/sbd/publicsite/index.aspx).

Weight Watchers

Weight Watchers organization is one of the oldest nutritional programs, dating back to the early 1960s. It is a weight reduction plan that teaches participants how to make better food choices and use portion control. There are no forbidden foods or restrictions but plenty of suggestions for creating a healthy eating environment and balancing food intake with exercise. A four-pillar scientific foundation was created using 45 years of trial and error and includes food, behavior, support, and exercise that can be incorporated into any lifestyle. If counseling a patient on this diet, it would be important to consider following suggestions for portion control and have a list of foods and point value for each. (http://www.weightwatchers.com/plan/index.aspx).

FOOD SAFETY AND PREPARATION

Even though your kitchen may rival that of an interior showplace, it may not be fit for cooking. Clean floors, spotless countertops, and organized cupboards are not indicators of a kitchen that employs "**safe food-handling** practices." We are unable to see, feel, or smell bacteria that contaminate our food. Keeping food safe for consumption depends on how it is stored, handled, and cooked. Eating food that contains harmful bacteria, toxins, parasites, viruses, or chemical contaminants can causes food-borne illness.

Campylobacter, Salmonella, Listeria, and *Escherichia coli* are the most common invaders. You do not have to eat a lot of contaminated food before you feel ill—you can become sick by eating just a few bites. Because **food-borne illnesses** resemble the common flu, many people are unaware it was the food that made them sick. Symptoms can appear about 30 minutes after eating or can take up to 3 weeks to manifest. It is estimated that up to 33 million people in the United States are sickened each year with a food-borne illness. To ensure that you are not part of this statistic, follow these four simple steps when handling or preparing food, which are highlighted in Food for Thought 11-6:

1. Clean
    a. Wash your hands for 20 seconds with hot, soapy water before and after handling food and after using the bathroom, playing with your pet, or changing diapers.
    b. Wash cutting boards, dishes, utensils, and countertops with hot, soapy water each time you prepare a new food for the meal. Food for Thought 11-7 gives advice for handling cutting boards.
    c. Use disposable paper towels versus cloth towels, which can harbor bacteria.
    d. Clean liquids that spill in the refrigerator, including those that leak out of packaged lunchmeat and hot dogs.
2. Separate (do not cross-contaminate)
    a. Separate raw meat, poultry, and seafood from other foods in your shopping cart and refrigerator and on the counter.
    b. Designate separate cutting boards for food groups: one for cutting meat, another for chopping vegetables, and another for slicing bread.
    c. Wash anything that comes into contact with raw meats and their juices with hot, soapy water.
    d. Use one plate for raw meat, poultry, and seafood and another plate after they are cooked.
3. Cook
    a. Use a thermometer to determine that food is fully cooked.
    b. Cook roasts and steaks to 145°C, poultry to 180°C, and pork to 160°C.
    c. Fish is done when it flakes with a fork.
    d. Never use or eat ground beef that is still pink.
    e. Cook eggs until both the yolk and white are firm, and avoid recipes that call for raw eggs. Food for Thought 11-8 provides further egg safety tips.
    f. Microwaved food should be hot throughout with no cold spots.
    g. Reheated food should be cooked to 165°C or boiled.
4. Chill
    a. Keep the temperature of your refrigerator at or below 41°C to slow the growth of bacteria.

b. Refrigerate or freeze perishables, cooked food, and all leftovers within 2 hours and put a date on the container. Leftovers should be used within 3 to 5 days.

c. Thaw food in the refrigerator, under cold water, or in the microwave—never on a counter at room temperature.

d. Marinate all food in the refrigerator.

e. Store leftovers in small shallow containers versus large containers for quick cooling.

f. Do not overpack the refrigerator—cool air must circulate to keep food safe.

🍎 FOOD FOR THOUGHT 11-6

FOUR STEPS OF FOOD SAFETY

1. Clean
2. Separate
3. Cook
4. Chill

🍎 FOOD FOR THOUGHT 11-7

CUTTING BOARD TIPS

- Use smooth cutting boards made of hard wood or plastic.
- Use one board for cutting meats and one for ready-to-eat foods such as vegetables, fruits, and bread.
- Boards should be free of cracks and crevices.
- Scrub boards with a brush in hot soapy water after use.
- Sanitize boards in the dishwasher or rinse in a solution of 1 teaspoon bleach in 1 quart of water.

🍎 FOOD FOR THOUGHT 11-8

EGG SAFETY TIPS

- Commercial products are made with pasteurized eggs that have been heated sufficiently to kill bacteria, or they contain an acidifying agent that kills bacteria.
- Commercial cookie dough is safe to eat uncooked.
- Buy only refrigerated eggs and keep them cold until ready to cook or serve.
- Cook eggs until they no longer run or scramble eggs until there is no visible liquid.

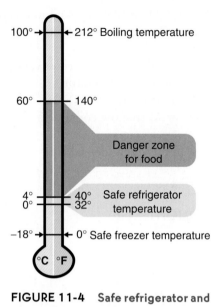

FIGURE 11-4   Safe refrigerator and freezer temperatures.

Figure 11-4 illustrates safe refrigeration temperatures and the danger zone for food.

OTHER KITCHEN DANGERS

Other **kitchen dangers** include lead, microwave packaging, and insects and dirt:

- Lead leached from ceramic dishes into food and drink is the number one source of dietary lead. To reduce your exposure to lead, do not use ceramic or lead crystal containers to store food. Use them sparingly for serving.
- Microwaving can cause adhesives and polymers from the package to leach into food. If at all possible, do not use the package carton to heat your food; instead, use a microwave-safe dish.
- Wash the tops of cans before removing lids to eliminate dust and dirt from falling into the food.
- Avoid storing food in cupboards under the sink or where water can leak or drain. Insects and rodents are attracted to dark, damp places and can invade openings in packages. Food for Thought 11-9 highlights safe kitchen tips and Food for Thought 11-10 suggests ways to keep vegetables safe.

🍎 **FOOD FOR THOUGHT 11-9**

TIPS FOR KEEPING A SAFE KITCHEN

- Keep dishcloths and sponges clean and dry. When wet, they harbor bacteria and promote bacterial growth.
- When washing dishes by hand, wash within 2 hours and air-dry so they are not handled when wet.
- If you have an infection or cut on your hands, wear rubber gloves and wash the gloves as often as bare hands.
- When thawing food in cold water, seal it in a water-tight bag and submerge it in water, changing the water every 30 minutes.
- Food defrosted in the microwave should be cooked immediately.
- Do not buy frozen seafood if the package is open, torn, or crushed on the edges.

🍎 **FOOD FOR THOUGHT 11-10**

KEEPING VEGETABLES SAFE

1. Do not buy vegetables that are bruised or damaged
2. Avoid precut vegetables or packaged salads that are not refrigerated
3. Wash your hands for 20 seconds before and after handling vegetables
4. Using soap and water, clean all surfaces and utensils used before and after preparing vegetables
5. Rinse all vegetables under cold running water for 2 minutes before cutting since bacteria can be transported to the flesh
6. Scrub the skin of root vegetables such as potatoes and carrots with a brush under cold running water
7. Wash bagged salads and precut vegetables even if the package says "ready to eat"
8. Cook sprouts before using them in recipes as bacteria grows inside sprouts
9. Keep vegetables away from raw meat, seafood, and poultry even when in the shopping cart, refrigerator, and on the counter
10. Refrigerate all cut, peeled, and cooked vegetables within 2 hours.

   Taken from Johns Hopkins Health Alert

COUNSELING PATIENTS

Sticking to the tried-and-true food guidelines are best when recommending a starting place for changing how your patient eats. Just as it is recommended that dental professionals only recommend products approved by the American Dental Association, we should suggest behaviors recommended by the Food Guidelines for Americans and the USDA Food Pyramid (or those from the patient's homeland). After collecting data and analyzing a food diary, do the following:

1. Compare the patient's food diary to suggestions made by MyPyramid or other food guide that would be best suited to his or her diet and cultural considerations, and point out excesses and deficiencies.
2. Choose food guidelines best suited to your patient's diet, medical and cultural tendencies, and suggest ways to improve in areas of neglect.
3. Recommend 30 minutes of moderate exercise each day, and work with your patient to discover ways to incorporate more movement into the daily schedule.
4. Outline safe food-handling and preparation techniques to ensure your patient is keeping food safe to prevent food-borne illnesses.

🍎 FOOD FOR THOUGHT 11-11

- Virginia Tech food researchers have provided significant evidence that visible wavelength of light cause taste and odor changes of food. The same ultraviolet rays that damage skin can also damage the nutritional value of food, so it is important to keep light out of food packages. Visible light degrades riboflavin in milk and interacts with flavor and odor molecules, so it is better to purchase milk in an opaque container for longer shelf life.[1]

- Some families have been stock piling food in the event of a national emergency. How do we know which foods will store well and last for years? Even though a food product may have a "best if used by" date on its package, it may still be palatable and OK to eat in an emergency situation, according to food researchers at Brigham Young University. Sugar and salt can be stored indefinitely and other dry goods such as cereal grains, dry milk, and rice, stored in containers, can be kept for decades as long as they are properly sealed and away from moisture, heat, and light.[2]

- The 5-second rule surmises that your dropped food will still be germ-free if retrieved from a dirty floor or surface within 5 seconds. If you live and work in a sanitized environment, chances of the dropped food picking up bacteria would be slim. Moist sticky food makes more contact with a surface so it would pick up more bacteria than dry food. If only a few "germs" stick to the food, a healthy immune system can

Continued on next page

fight off infection. But if you drop your food in a germ-infested area, it is a sure thing you will get sick. So if the surface looks or smells bad, forget the 5-second rule and throw out the food.[3]

- Just how clean are the restaurant plates you eat off of? According to food scientists at Ohio State University, looking clean is not enough. Washing technique should be a 3-step process—scrub in soapy hot water at 110°F (uncomfortably hot), rinse with clean water, and then soak in a sanitizer. A lipstick mark on a cup is not necessarily a bad sign as it keeps bacteria from sticking. And silverware utensils are actually better breeding grounds for bacteria than ceramic plates. Next time you visit your favorite restaurant, casually ask if they soak their plates in a sanitizer.[4]

- Chemists at University of South Carolina have invented dipsticks made of polymer that can be carried to restaurants, grocery stores, or used at home that detect the presence of biologic amines that cause food spoilage. Not all spoiled food looks weird, grows mold, or smells bad, so spoilage can be hard to detect. The polymer dipstick will change color depending on the degree of spoilage, allowing the consumer to make a choice "to eat or not to eat."[5]

- Duke University and Arizona State University researchers suggest that when disgusting products touch other products in the shopping cart, or on store shelves, consumers are less likely to want to eat or use the item. Products identified as disgusting were trash bags, cat litter, diapers, feminine napkins, cigarettes, mayonnaise, and shortening. Study participants were less likely to desire a cookie after seeing the package touch feminine napkins. Rice cakes in clear packaging touching lard were perceived as having higher fat content than rice cakes in opaque packaging. Store displays should take into account neighboring products that are surrounding, touching, or in clear packaging.[6]

1. Virginia Tech (2007, August 27). Food packaging that provides visibility can reduce shelf life. Science Daily. (www.sciencedaily.com/releases/2007/08)
2. Brigham Young University. Keeping food for years and certain dry foods are good past their best-before date, food scientists say. Science Daily (www.sciencedaily.com/videos/2007/0208)
3. University of Wisconsin, Madison (2007, September 29). Is there any validity to the so-called 5-second rule? Science Daily. (www.sciencedaily.com/releases/2007/08)
4. Ohio State University. Are your dishes clean? What kills *E. coli* and *salmonella* bacteria? Science Daily (www.sciencedaily.com/videos/2007/0810)
5. American Chemical Society (2007, April 2) chemists are creating an easy-home test kit for spoiled food. Science Daily (www.sciencedaily.com/releases/2007/03/070326095846.htm)
6. Duke University (2007, May 3) When cookies catch the cooties. Science Daily (www.sciencedaily.con/releases/2007/04/070430155728.htm)

Putting This Into Practice

1. Using the guidelines from around the world, for example, invent a 10-point dietary guidelines to lead your family into a healthier lifestyle.
2. Explain the key differences between MyPyramid for adults and for children.
3. Make a food pyramid or other shape to illustrate your family's current eating habits, including favorite foods cut from magazines.
4. Using your family's food pyramid, list some changes that should be made to follow the dietary guidelines you developed for your family.

WEB RESOURCES

Easy Ways to Keep Vegetables Safe http://www.johnshopkinshealthalerts.com/alerts/nutrition_weight_control/JohnsHopkinsNutritionandWeightControlHealthAlert_1150-1.html?st=email&s=ENH%20070919%20013

Partnership for Food Safety Education—Fight Bac!: Keep Food Safe From Bacteria www.fightbac.org

Dietary Guidelines for Americans http://www.health.gov/DietaryGuidelines/

Canada's Food Guide http://www.hc-sc.gc.ca/fn-an/food-guide-aliment/index_e.html

2002 American Dietetic Association – Comparison of International Food Guides – Pictorial Representation http://www.senba.es/recursos/piramides/pictorials_nutrition_guides.pdf

German Nutrition Society www.iuns.org/adhering-bodies/report/germany.htm

MyPyramid for Kids No Junk Food in Public Schools http://www.nojunkfood.org/policy/ http://www.mypyramid.gov/kids/index.html

Vegan Food Pyramid http://www.chooseveg.com/vegan-food-pyramid.asp

American Institute for Cancer Research: Food, Nutrition, Physical Activity, and the Prevention of Cancer http://www.dietandcancerreport.org/

European Food information Council http://www.eufic.org/index/en/

Food Safety—Gateway to Government Food Safety Information www.foodsafety.gov

U.S. Food and Drug Administration—Center for Food Safety and Applied Nutrition http://vm.cfsan.fda.gov/

U.S. Food and Drug Administration www.fda.gov

U.S. Department of Health and Human Services—The Surgeon General's Call to Action to Prevent and Decrease Overweight and Obesity www.surgeongeneral.gov/topics/obesity

Harvard School of Public Health—Food Pyramids www.hsph.harvard.edu/nutritionsource/pyramids.html

American Dietetic Association www.eatright.org

Federal Citizen Information Center www.pueblo.gsa.gov

Vegetarian Food Pyramid www.vegsource.com/nutrition/pyramid.htm

Food and Nutrition Information Center www.nal.usda.gov/fnic/Fpyr/pyramid.html

The British Dietetic Association http://cgi.www.bda.uk.com/

For more information about safe food handling and preparation:

1. USDA's Meat and Poultry Hotline: 1-800-535-4555
2. FDA's Food Information and Seafood Hotline: 1-800-332-4010

REFERENCES

1. Reedy J, Krebs-Smith SM. A comparison of food based recommendations and nutrient values of three food guides: USDA's MyPyramid, NHLBI's dietary approaches to stop hypertension eating plan, and Hardard's healthy eating pyramid. *J Am diet Assoc* 2008;108(3):522–528.
2. Lichtenstein AH, Rasmussen H, Yu WW, et al. Modified MyPyramid for older adults. *J Nutr* 2008;138(1):5–11.
3. Kranz S, Lin PJ, Wagstaff DA. Children's dairy intake in the United States: too little, too fat? *J Pediatr* 2007;151(6):642–646.
4. Chiuve SE, Willett WC. The 2005 food guide pyramid: an opportunity lost? *Nat Clin Pract Cardiovasc Med* 2007;4(11):610–620.
5. Krebs-Smith SM, Kris-Etherton P. How does MyPyramid compare to other population based recommendations for controlling chronic disease? *J Am Diet Assoc* 2007; 107(5):830–837.
6. Guenther PM, Dodd KW, Reedy J, et al. Most Americans eat much less than recommended amounts of fruits and vegetables. *J Am Diet Assoc* 2006;106(9):1371–1379.
7. Marshall TA. Dietary guidelines for Americans and MyPyramid. *J Am Dent Assoc* 2006;137(9):1344.

SUGGESTED READING

Almanza BA, Namkung Y, Ismail JA, et al. Client's safe food handling knowledge and risk behaviors in a home-delivered meal program. *J Am Diet Assoc* 2007;107(5):816–821.

Centers for Disease Control and Prevention. Preliminary foodnet data on the incidence of infection with pathogens transmitted commonly through food-10 states, United States, 2005, *MMWR Morb Mortal Wkly Rep* 2006;55(14):392–395.

Chittick P, Sulka A, Tauxe RV, et al. A summary of national reports of food-borne outbreaks of Salmonella Heidelberg infections in the United States: clues for disease prevention. *J Food Prot* 2006;69(5):1150–1153.

Jones TF, Angulo FJ. Eating in restaurants: a risk factor for food-borne disease? *Clin Infect Dis* 2006;43(10):132–138.

Kendall PA, Hillers VV, Medeiros LC. Food safety guidance for older adults. *Clin Infect Dis* 2006;42(9):1298–1304.

Stegeman C, Kunselman B, McClure E, et al. *Fad diets: implications for oral health care treatment*. 2006;30–35.

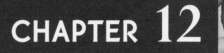

CHAPTER 12

READING LABELS

OBJECTIVES

Upon completion of the chapter, the reader will be able to:

1 Outline the major points of the Nutrition Labeling and Education Act (NLEA)
2 Discuss the importance of including trans fats on Nutrition Facts labels
3 List nutrients that must be included on a food label
4 Explain the meaning of Daily Value (DV) on a food label
5 Describe how food ingredients are listed
6 Give examples of health claims
7 State five common mistakes when reading a food label
8 Identify the number of calories per gram for carbohydrates, protein, fat, and alcohol
9 Calculate the percentage of a given nutrient in a food product and the amount of calories in a serving of food product

KEY TERMS

100% Natural	Low Carbohydrate	Nutrition Facts
Daily Value	Kilocalorie	Organic Food Products
Health Claims	NLEA	Trans Fat

In 1990, the U.S. Food and Drug Administration (FDA) established the Nutrition Labeling and Education Act (**NLEA**) to help consumers know what they are buying so that they can make healthier food and snack selections. The NLEA requires food package labels for all food except meat and poultry, and is voluntary for raw produce and fish. The NLEA also set guidelines for stating nutrient claims, such as "low-fat" or "sugar-free," and certain FDA-approved health claims, such as "lowers cholesterol." Learning to read a food label is like learning a specialized lingo. Just as you had to learn to use dental terminology, you also have to learn nutritional terminology. All food labels are titled "Nutrition Facts" and contain the same information, allowing consumers to compare similar products and to calculate the amount of nutrients consumed daily. In 1994, food package labeling became law. The following foods are exceptions to that law and do not require food labels:

- Food served in hospital cafeterias, on airplanes, in vending machines, and at mall counters
- Bakery, deli, or candy store that serves ready-to-eat food prepared on site
- Food shipped in bulk
- Medical foods that are consumed to address the needs of certain diseases
- Coffee, tea, spices, or other nonnutritive foods
- Food served in restaurants, unless they make a health or nutrient claim on their menu, advertisement, or other notice

An American Dietetics Association survey revealed that 71% of Americans read labels, but that most become confused while doing so. Learning to separate fact from fiction is necessary to accurately read a label and to make good choices when purchasing food. Although labels are not meant to be tricky, they can be misleading if not read carefully. It is important to check food labels even if you are a routine shopper because just as the design of a food product label can change, so can the ingredients. Routine shoppers have a tendency to make the same food choices, like the same brand of baked beans or loaf of bread each time they need baked beans or bread. Manufacturers can change ingredients at any given time, and unless the label is read and compared to other like products, there is no guarantee you are making the healthiest food choice.

READING A NUTRITION FACTS LABEL

There are many reasons for reading a label other than to know what ingredients the product contains or whether it is "rich" in certain nutrients. Individuals following a specific diet might need to know how much fat or carbohydrates a product has. "**Nutrition Facts**" contain several parts and under the NLEA, food manufacturers are *required* to provide daily values, based on a 2,000-calorie diet, for the following:

- Total calories
- Calories from fat
- Calories from saturated fat
- Total fat
- Polyunsaturated fat
- Saturated fat
- Trans fat (new)
- Monounsaturated fat
- Cholesterol
- Sodium
- Potassium
- Total carbohydrate
- Dietary fiber
- Soluble fiber
- Insoluble fibers
- Sugars
- Sugar alcohols
- Protein
- Vitamin A
- Percentage of vitamin A as beta-carotene
- Vitamin C
- Calcium
- Iron
- Other added nutrients

Figure 12-1 provides an example of a typical food label.

Serving sizes, listed at the top under the title, have long been an issue with nutritionists when a package that appears to be one serving may actually be two or two-and-a-half, as with a 20-oz soda. When you eat a whole box of macaroni and cheese or a can of soup, it may be two servings, yet the information on the label is for one serving. That means all nutrient values should be multiplied by two. Figure 12-2 compares value for two servings versus one.

The percentage **Daily Value** (DV) column helps you figure how much of a nutrient you are getting from a food that contributes to your total daily intake. If a label has 25% for vitamin A, it means you have to accumulate 75% from other food the rest of the day to reach 100% of the recommended intake. Sodium, saturated

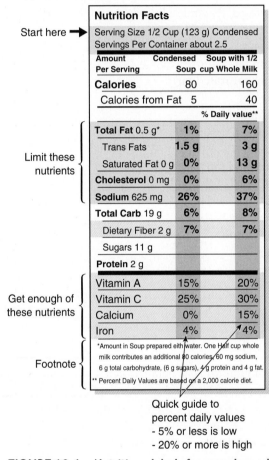

FIGURE 12-1 Nutrition label for condensed tomato soup.

fat, and sugars are the three listed nutrients you want to keep track of to make sure you are not getting more than you need. Excess of these three may lead to serious heart problems, hypertension, and obesity.

Calories per serving appear on the label under serving size. It is important to know how many calories per day you eat to compute your DV of nutrients. Although the labels are based on a 2,000-calorie diet, as explained at the bottom in the footnote, it is recommended that women in the age-group of 35 to 70 restrict their diet to 1,600 to 1,800 calories per day, and men in the same age-group

Example					
	Single serving	Percentage DV		Double serving	Percentage DV
Serving size	1 cup (228 g)			2 cups (456 g)	
Calories	250			500	
Calories from fat	110			220	
Total fat	12 g	18%		24 g	36%
Trans fat	1.5 g			3 g	
Saturated fat	3 g	15%		6 g	30%
Cholesterol	30 mg	10%		60 mg	20%
Sodium	470 mg	20%		940 mg	50%
Total carbohydrate	31 g	10%		62 g	20%
Dietary fiber	0 g	0%		0 g	0%
Sugars	5 g			10 g	
Protein	5 g			10 g	
Vitamin A		4%			8%
Vitamin C		2%			4%
Calcium		20%			40%
Iron		4%			8%

FIGURE 12-2 Comparison of two labels showing calculations for consuming two servings.

consume 2,000 to 2,200 calories per day.[1] Depending on whether you are male or female and active or sedentary, you may have to increase or decrease the rest of the day's nutrients. Computing the DV for nutrients would then require a good pair of reading glasses and a calculator.

Trans fats are the newest addition to Nutrition Facts labels. FDA estimates that the average person eats 4.7 lbs of trans fats per year. A small amount of **trans fat** is naturally occuring in beef and dairy products, but most of the trans fat in our diets comes from infusing vegetable oils with hydrogen. Manufacturers began using hydrogenated fats about 20 years ago to prolong the shelf-life of their product. If in fact, a Twinkie stays soft for years, it is no doubt due to the hydrogenated oil in its ingredients. We should minimize trans fats in our diets because they have the same effect on our arteries as bacon grease. According to reports from Mayo Clinic, trans fats are actually worse for us than saturated fats because not only do they clog arteries but are also bad for cholesterol levels—increases low-density lipoprotein (LDL) level and lowers high-density lipoprotein (HDL) level, which protects the heart. Food for Thought 12-1 details the history of eliminating trans fats from food.

🍎 FOOD FOR THOUGHT 12-1

An organization called "Ban Trans Fats" started an initiative in 2003 to ban trans fats from all food by suing Kraft to eliminate trans fats from the ubiquitous Oreo cookie. Not only did Kraft eliminate trans fats in its cookie but also eliminated it from more than 640 other foods it manufactured. The law suit, through media attention, created intense public interest in the perils of trans fat which created a chain reaction in the food manufacturing industry. Once it started, there was no turning back. Visit their website at: http://www.bantransfats.com/

In past years, the only way to determine if a food product contained trans fats was to read the ingredients and look for the word hydrogenated as their value was not listed along with other fats on labels. The Center for Science in the Public Interest (CSPI), a consumer watch-dog group, became alarmed by the news that trans fats were unhealthy for the heart but were hidden on food labels. In 1993, the CSPI began to lobby the FDA to require trans fats on nutrition labels. After 10 years of unrelenting pressure, the FDA mandated that, as of January 2006, all labels will indicate amount of trans fat under the line for saturated fat. There is no Daily Value recommended but it is important to add the amount of trans fat to amount of saturated fat. A combined amount under 5% total DV is desirable. Table 12-1 indicates major food sources of trans fats.

Food for Thought 12-2 details daily supplements which may have trace amounts of trans fats.

🍎 FOOD FOR THOUGHT 12-2

Dietary supplements may contain trans fats if partially hydrogenated vegetable oil is used in the manufacturing process. If the product contains 0.5 g or more of trans fat, manufacturers must include it on the Supplements Facts panel.

TABLE 12-1	Trans Fat in Common Foods
Food	Approximate Grams of Trans Fat
Crackers	0.36 g per crackers
Pound cake	4.3 g per slice
Cream-filled cookies	1.9 g each
Microwave popcorn	5 g per half bag
KFC original recipe chicken dinner	7 g
Doughnuts	5 g each
Potato chips	3 g small bag
French fries	10 g medium serving
Maria Calendar's chicken pot pie	1.96 g
Mrs. Smith's apple pie	4 g each slice
Nabisco chips ahoy	1.5 g per 3
Stick margarine	2.8 g per tablespoon

KFC, Kentucky Fried Chicken.

INGREDIENTS

Ingredients are listed from the most abundant ingredient to the least abundant. For example, on a loaf of bread, you would assume the first ingredient listed would be bread flour, or beans on a can of green beans. Two facts are very important to remember when looking at this section, because there are two ingredients that may appear to be "hidden":

1. Sugars are sometimes listed separately, but if added together would be the first ingredient. Food for Thought 12-3 lists other names for sugar.
2. Anything partially hydrogenated affects the body the same way as saturated fat. Food for Thought 12-4 lists examples of trans fats.

🍎 **FOOD FOR THOUGHT 12-3**

HIDDEN SUGAR

Brown sugar	Invert sugar
Corn sweetener	Lactose
Corn syrup	Malt syrup
Dextrose	Maltose
Fructose	Molasses
Fruit juice concentrate	Raw sugar
Glucose	Sucrose
High-fructose corn syrup	Syrup
Honey	Turbinado sugar

🍎 **FOOD FOR THOUGHT 12-4**

TRANS FATS

Partially hydrogenated corn oil
Partially hydrogenated soybean oil
Partially hydrogenated cottonseed oil
Fully hydrogenated vegetable oil

HEALTH CLAIMS

Health claims are posted on the front of the food package to entice shoppers looking for a certain benefit from their food. The NLEA specifies which claims are allowed and the requirements the food has to meet to make that claim. Do not make the mistake that "fat-free" foods are "calorie-free." Manufacturers usually increase the sugar content of fat-free foods to make up for what is lost by reducing the fat content. The texture of fat is lost but the taste is not compromised. Table 12-2 explains the FDA requirements that must be met to make certain health claims, and Table 12-3 explains the meaning of certain health claims.

Organic

To use the word **organic** on a label, a food grower must prove that he or she was able to produce the food in a way that was good for the earth. Ninety-five percent

TABLE 12-2 U.S. Food and Drug Administration (FDA) Requirements to Meet Health Claims

Health Claim	Requirements to Meet
Fat-free	0.5 g of fat per serving or less
0 g Trans fat	<0.5 g of trans fat per serving
Low-fat	3 g of fat per serving or less
Less fat	25% less fat than original recipe
Light (fat)	50% less fat than original recipe
Saturated fat-free	0.5 g of saturated or trans fat per serving or less
Cholesterol-free	2 g or less saturated fat/serving and <2 mg cholesterol per serving
Low cholesterol	2 g or less saturated fat/serving and <20 mg cholesterol per serving
Reduced calorie	25% fewer calories than original recipe
Low calorie	40 calories or less per serving
Light (calories)	One third fewer calories than original recipe
Extra lean	5 g fat or less, 2 g saturated fat or less, 95 mg cholesterol/100 g serving of meat, poultry, or seafood
Lean	10 g fat or less, 4.5 g saturated fat or less, 95 mg cholesterol/100 g serving of meat, poultry, or seafood
High fiber	5 g or more per serving
Sugar-free	0.5 g or less per serving
Sodium-free (salt-free)	0.5 g or less per serving
Low sodium	140 mg or less per serving
Very low sodium	35 mg or less per serving
Heart Healthy	Low in saturated fat, cholesterol, sodium

TABLE 12-3	Meanings of Health Claims
Health Claim	**Meaning**
Healthy	Low in fat, saturated fat, cholesterol, and sodium and has at least 10% DV of protein, iron, calcium, fiber, and vitamins A and C
Good source of, more, added	10% more DV of given nutrients than original recipe
High, rich in, excellent source of	20% or more of the given nutrient per serving
Less, fewer, reduced	25% less of given nutrients than original recipe
Low, little, few, low source of	Frequent consumption of food will not exceed DV

DV, daily value.

of the ingredients used in the process must have been organic, which means that the food was nurtured without synthetic pesticides, fertilizers, antibiotics, hormones, or genetic engineering. Organic food products usually cost more than nonorganic counterparts because the process is more labor intensive and requires more time from field to market. There are fewer growing opportunities during a season and harvests can be smaller. Organic crops are rotated and so soil is not nutrient depleted and plants are grown without chemical fertilizers. Therefore, more hand weeding is needed. Organic crops grown as livestock feed are more expensive than nonorganic and so the cost for meat from organically nurtured animals is also passed on to the consumer. Even so, some consumers feel the extra cost to buy organic food products is worth the peace of mind, knowing that there are no chemicals mixed in with the food and that the earth was treated as gently as possible.

100% Natural

Sometimes the terms **100% Natural** and "organic" are mistakenly used to mean the same thing. But the claim of 100% natural is meant to reveal that there are no artificial colors, flavors, or preservatives in the food product. 100% Natural does not necessarily mean the food product is good for you because it could be loaded with sugar and fat. Empty calorie foods can be all natural but bad for your diet and contribute very little to your daily nutrient value. Years ago 7-Up was marketed as 100% Natural, and although it may have had natural flavorings, it was not the best nutritious beverage choice.

Low Carbohydrate

This claim on food has no current standard, so it can mean whatever the food manufacturer wants it to mean. It became important during the popularity of the Atkins Diet which suggested eliminating carbohydrates from the diet. Those looking for this claim should make sure they read the label because often manufacturers will replace carbohydrates with high-fat ingredients, sugar alcohols, or artificial sweeteners. Calorie-wise, the food can contain as many calories as the same product that is not low carbohydrate.

No Antibiotics

This claim is seen on packages of meat, poultry, and milk to indicate that the animals were raised without routinely using antibiotics to keep them healthy while growing. Approximately 11 million kg of antibiotics are fed to U.S. livestock each year. In a U.S. Department of Agriculture (USDA)-funded study conducted at the University of Minnesota, scientists found antibiotic residue in plants that were grown using manure excreted by animals that were fed antibiotics.[2] This means that organic farmers can only use the manure from livestock that were not fed antibiotics, adding to the reasons why organic produce costs more.

No Hormones

This health claim is seen on beef and dairy product labels when the animals were raised without administering hormones. Food products with this label cost more than their counterparts because it takes longer to get the product to market. Hormones can cause a rapid growth cycle which means less time between birth and slaughter, and that means feed costs are reduced. And when dairy cows are fed hormones, it causes them to produce more milk. There are six USDA-approved female growth hormones and a recombinant bovine growth hormone (rbGH) for faster milk production. Accusations have been made that the growth hormones fed to cattle and dairy cows end up in the food we eat and cause our children to reach puberty at an earlier age, but there are no definitive studies to prove this.

Food for Thought 12-5 lists words that are not FDA approved as health claims.

🍎 **FOOD FOR THOUGHT 12-5**

The words right, smart, and natural are not FDA approved as health claims.

COMMON MISTAKES WHEN READING LABELS

There are five common mistakes made when reading labels.

1. Not reading serving sizes. A can of soup is usually two or two-and-a-half servings, so all values must be multiplied accordingly.
2. Forgetting that all label values are based on a 2,000-calorie diet. If you eat fewer or more than 2,000 calories, an adjustment must be made.
3. Thinking "reduced-fat" or "reduced sodium" on the label means the food is low fat or low sodium. All it means is that the food has 25% less fat or sodium. If the amount of either was high to begin with, reducing by 25% would not make much of a difference.
4. Thinking the percentage of DV is the percentage of calories. If the DV is 20%, it means you have consumed 20% of the recommended nutrient for the day.
5. Assuming the amount of sugar on a label is all added sugar. If one of the ingredients naturally has sugar, such as an orange, the amount of sugar includes what the ingredient naturally brings to the product.

FOOD ENERGY = CALORIES

The word **kilocalorie**, shortened to kcal, is the correct way to refer to the energy produced by food and expended by our bodies, although it is more commonly referred to as *calorie*. Most food has a calorie value, or the ability to provide energy. Knowing how many calories per gram a nutrient provides is the first step in "figuring nutrient" (instead of doing the) calculations. The following are calorie values of three major nutrients plus alcohol:

- Carbohydrates: 4 cal/g
- Protein: 4 cal/g
- Fat: 9 cal/g
- Alcohol: 7 cal/g

CALCULATIONS

When working with numbers, you have to use similar values to multiply or divide. This means to find percentage of calories, both numbers have to be calories. One cannot be grams and the other calories.

To compute the number of calories from grams:

1. Find the number of grams of the nutrient.
2. Multiply by 4 for carbohydrate or protein, or 9 for fat.
3. Your answer is the number of calories generated from the nutrient.

Example:

If there are 32 g of carbohydrate: 4×32 g $= 128$ calories.
If there are 14 g of fat: 9×14 g $= 126$ calories.

Food for Thought 12-6 lists caloric values for major nutrients.

🍎 FOOD FOR THOUGHT 12-6

USE THE FOLLOWING VALUES WHEN COMPUTING THE NUMBER OF CALORIES FROM GRAMS

Carbohydrate (CHO) 4 cal/g
Protein 4 cal/g
Fat 9 cal/g
Alcohol 7 cal/g

Fat is the primary nutrient that is restricted in daily diets, and the one that is usually factored from a label to determine if the food product is a healthy choice. To keep track of how much fat you have in your diet, computing the percentage of calories that come from fat in a food will help you decide if it is something you want to include in your meal.

1. Find the total number of calories for a serving size.
2. Find the total number of calories from fat.
3. Divide the calories from fat by the total calories and multiply by 100 to get a percentage.
4. If it is more than 30%, it is probably not a good choice.

COUNSELING PATIENTS

Reading labels is a learned skill. Teaching your patient how to read labels and how the information can work to improve the food choices can have a great impact on long-term health. The following are some suggestions when teaching your patients this important tool for food selection:

1. Suggest that they bring in labels from the following:
   a. Packages of their favorite foods
   b. Packages of similar foods for comparison
2. Calculate a healthy range for calories consumed daily, taking into consideration the following factors:
   a. Age
   b. Body size
   c. Desired weight
   d. Activity level
3. Identify the parts of the label for them:
   a. Serving size: point out that some containers have more than one serving size
   b. Total calories per serving and those from fat
   c. DV of nutrient values
   d. Ingredients: instruct about:
      i. Hidden sugars
      ii. Trans fats
   e. Footnote: values are based on a 2,000-calorie diet
4. Explain the meaning of certain health claims.
5. Identify which nutrients are most important to your patient and explain how to obtain the percentage contained in a serving size.
6. Review common mistakes when reading labels.

Putting This Into Practice

1. If one serving of baked beans has 260 calories and the label says there are 2 g of fat per serving, how many calories are from fat?
2. If one serving of Toaster Strudel has 350 calories and 140 of those calories are from fat, what percentage of the Toaster Strudel is fat?

(continued)

3. If one cup of Cranapple juice has 160 calories with 30 g of carbohydrates, what percentage of the calories are carbohydrates?

4. There are 1.5 g of protein in one serving of Campbell's beef and potato soup. The can has two servings but you eat the whole can. How many grams of protein have you consumed?

5. If one serving of turkey breast has 60 calories and the label says that there are 1.5 g of fat per serving, how many calories are from fat?

6. If one serving of turkey breast has 60 calories with 13.5 of those calories being fat, what percentage of the turkey breast is fat?

7. If one cup of Instant Breakfast has 250 calories with 30 g being carbohydrates, what percentage of the Instant Breakfast is carbohydrate?

8. Compare labels for Campbell's and Healthy Choice chicken noodle soup. Which contains the most sodium per serving?

9. If a label states the DV for vitamin A is 25%, how much of the vitamin do you need to consume in other foods throughout the day? (See RDI in Chapter 5)

WEB RESOURCES

FDA: How to Understand and Use the Nutrition Facts Label
http://www.cfsan.fda.gov/~dms/foodlab.html

FDA: Trans Fatty Acids in Nutrition Labeling http://www.cfsan.fda.gov/~dms/transgui.html

Center for Science in the Public Interest: Trans Fats http://www.cspinet.org/transfat/

FDA Fact Sheet: What Every Consumer Should Know About Trans Fats
http://www.fda.gov/oc/initiatives/transfat/q_a.html

FDA: Trans Fats Now Listed With Saturated Fat and Cholesterol on Food Labels
http://www.cfsan.fda.gov/~dms/transfat.html

Nutrition Facts for Fast Food http://www.fatcalories.com/

REFERENCES

1. Burros M. *US Diet Proposals Reflect Nation's Lack of Fitness*. New York Times; 2003.
2. Holly Dolliver, Kuldip Kumar, Satish Gupta. Sulfamethazine uptake by plants from manure-amended soil. *J Environ Qual* 2007;36:1224–1230.

SUGGESTED READING

Department of Health and Human Services, Food and Drug Administration. Food labeling: trans fatty acids in nutrition labeling, nutrient content claims, and health claims. *Final rule. Fed Regist* 2003;68(133):41433–41506.

PART V

FOOD FOR GROWTH

CHAPTER 13

NUTRIENT NEEDS FOR DEVELOPMENT, GROWTH, AND MAINTENANCE OF ORAL STRUCTURES

OBJECTIVES

Upon completion of this chapter, the reader will be able to:

1 Explain the difference between preeruptive nutrition and posteruptive nutrition
2 Give examples of preeruptive and posteruptive effects of deficiencies in key nutrients
3 Define critical period and explain the need for good maternal nutrition for future oral health
4 List nutrients necessary for proper tooth calcification
5 Identify the nutrient necessary for development of healthy epithelial tissue and salivary gland function
6 List nutrients that assist with wound healing
7 Discuss the role fluoride plays preeruptively and posteruptively and explain the significance of ingestion of too much fluoride during the critical period

KEY TERMS

Critical Period   Preeruptive
Maternal Nutrition   Posteruptive

A well-educated, well-informed dental clinician can determine by a quick glance around the oral cavity whether a patient has been well nourished during three phases of life: fetal development, preeruption of permanent teeth, and posteruption of permanent teeth. The oral cavity is a treasure trove of information regarding past and present nutritional choices and habits.

EFFECTS OF DIET DURING THE CRITICAL PERIOD OF DEVELOPMENT

The **critical period** of development is the time during which the environment has the greatest impact on the developing embryo. The presence or absence of specific nutrients during fetal development can make the difference between health and disease of soft and hard structures. In the **preeruptive** stage, mineralization of primary teeth begins during the third or fourth month of pregnancy. At birth, crowns of primary teeth are almost completely formed, and by the age of 1 year, calcification of the crowns of permanent teeth is mostly completed. Well-formed, well-calcified tooth structure can reduce the incidences of dental caries later in the life cycle. Presence or lack of other nutrients can make the difference between high-functioning salivary glands or those that are atrophied and produce little saliva. It also can make the difference between periodontal tissues that are resistant to bacterial invasion or those that have a tendency to pocket formation. **Maternal nutrition** plays a critical role in the fetus developing healthy oral structures. Although we have no control over the nutrition habits of our biological mothers, **posteruptively**, we can learn to develop healthy nutritional habits to countereffect any deficiencies that resulted in poorly formed hard and soft structures. Table 13-1 provides a list of nutrients, structure affected, and functions in the oral cavity.

VITAMIN A

The general function of vitamin A is for synthesis of epithelial tissues.

- Preeruptively, vitamin A assists in the formation of mucous-secreting cells of the salivary glands and helps with the normal formation of enamel and dentin.
- Posteruptively, vitamin A maintains epithelial tissues and keeps the salivary glands working. It also maintains the integrity of the sulcular epithelium.

TABLE 13-1	Nutrients and Their Effects and Functions	
Nutrient	**Structure Affected**	**Other Function**
Fat-soluble vitamins		
Vitamin A	Salivary glands	—
	Sulcular epithelium	—
Vitamin D	Teeth—enamel, cementum	Calcification of all hard tissues
	Bone	—
Vitamin K	—	Blood clotting
Water-soluble vitamins		
Vitamin C	Collagen—dentin, pulp, cementum, alveolar bone, periodontal fibers, blood vessels, periodontal ligament	Wound healing
B Complex	Tongue, soft tissues	—
Cobalamine	—	—
Folacin	—	Deficiency may cause cleft lip and palate
Minerals		
Calcium	Enamel, cementum, bone	Calcification of all hard tissues
Phosphorus	Enamel, cementum, bone	Calcification of all hard tissues
Iron	—	Synthesis of hemoglobin
Zinc	—	Wound healing
Fluoride	Enamel	Strengthens enamel as it forms
Major nutrients		
Protein	Maxilla, mandible, periodontal tissues	Repair and maintenance of tissues

[handwritten annotation: Synthesis of epithelial tissues]

[handwritten annotation: Vit A Formation Synthesis of epithelial tissues salivary glands]

If there is a deficiency of vitamin A in the diet:

- Preeruptively, it could cause abnormal formation of enamel and dentin and contribute to the formation of cleft lip and/or palate and abnormal formation of salivary glands.
- Posteruptively, it could cause salivary glands to atrophy, reducing the amount of saliva available to the oral cavity. It could also hyperkeratinize normally thin, mucous membranes. Periodontal tissues can appear hyperkeratinized or hyperplastic with a tendency to pocket formation.

VITAMIN D

The general function of vitamin D is to enhance absorption of calcium and phosphorous.

- Preeruptively, it aids with the calcification of all hard tissues—bone, enamel, dentin, and cementum.
- Posteruptively, it helps repair diseased bone.

If there is a deficiency of vitamin D in the diet:

- Preeruptively, it could cause enamel or dentin hypoplasia.
- Posteruptively, it could cause osteomalacia in adults and loss of lamina dura, as seen on dental radiographs. A deficiency results in an overall lack of mineralization of bone and cementum.

VITAMIN K

Vitamin K aids with blood clotting time, so a deficiency of this nutrient could cause prolonged clotting time.

VITAMIN C

Vitamin C helps with formation of collagen, which includes dentin, pulp, cementum, alveolar bone, periodontal fibers, blood vessels, gingival nerves, and periodontal ligament.

- Preeruptively, it helps with formation of bone and teeth as well as formation of all connective tissues.
- Posteruptively, it helps with formation of collagen, wound healing, and formation of connective tissues. It maintains the integrity of blood vessels and assists with phagocytosis.

A long-term deficiency in vitamin C results in the deficiency disease of scurvy. Oral appearance of scurvy mocks advanced, acute periodontal disease. Gingival tissues appear dark red to purple, spongy, and hemorrhagic; teeth are mobile; and breath is fetid. Its diagnosis is unusual in developed countries, but it is seen on rare occasions. If there is a mild deficiency of vitamin C:

Vit C formation of collagen dentin, pulp, cementum

- Preeruptively, it can cause irregular formation or absence of dentin.
- Posteruptively, it can cause enlarged, bluish-red, hemorrhagic gingival tissues.

B COMPLEX VITAMINS

The B complex vitamins are coenzymes and work together to maintain healthy oral tissues. Deficiencies can be seen in the oral cavity:

Vit B healthy oral tissues effects tongue

- Deficiency of thiamin (vitamin B_1) can cause the deficiency disease of beriberi. There is an increase in the sensitivity of oral tissues. The tongue exhibits a burning sensation and there is a general loss of taste.
- Deficiency of niacin (vitamin B_3) can cause the deficiency disease of pellagra. It affects the tongue, causing it to be sore, red, and swollen. Pain with eating and swallowing accompanies the symptoms.
- Deficiency of riboflavin (vitamin B_2) also affects the tongue, causing it to be inflamed. It also causes angular chelosis, and a greasy, red, scaly lesion resembling a butterfly shape can develop around the nose.
- Deficiency of cobalamine (B_{12}) causes pernicious anemia and a bright red, smooth, burning tongue.
- Deficiency of folacin also causes a burning tongue and oral mucosa, angular chelosis, gingivitis, and frequent oral lesions. There has been much research about the relationship between lack of folic acid during fetal development and cleft lips and palates.

CALCIUM AND PHOSPHORUS

Calcium and phosphorus are needed in abundance for calcification of hard tissues and need vitamin D to help with absorption.

Vit D help w/absorption

- Preeruptively, they are responsible for mineralization of enamel, cementum, and bone.
- Posteruptively, they remineralize hard tissues and maintain bone.

If there is a deficiency of calcium and phosphorus in the diet:

- Preeruptively, it could cause hypocalcification of enamel.
- Posteruptively, it could allow bone loss.

bone loss

FLUORIDE

Fluoride is a unique nutritive substance in that it can be detrimental if too much or too little is ingested during the critical period of growth in the age-group of 6 months to 2.5 years when permanent teeth are developing. Too little fluoride during this period can result in the teeth being more susceptible to dental caries, and too much during this period can result in enamel fluorosis. There is an optimal level of ingestion that falls somewhere between too much and too little, but there are many factors to consider and various avenues of delivery that make it difficult to control: community water supply, fluoridated toothpaste, fluoride content in food and beverages, amount consumed, and stage of tooth development during consumption. Visit the American Dental Association website to learn more about their position on fluoride, recommended water levels, and supplementation schedule: http://www.ada.org/public/topics/fluoride/facts/fluoridation_facts.pdf

Preeruptively, it incorporates into the developing tooth structure to strengthen mineralizing tissues

Posteruptively, it continues to offer protective benefits against dental caries

If there is a deficiency of fluoride in the diet during tooth development:

- Preeruptively, calcified structures are weak, porous, and open for attack against acid destruction
- Posteruptively, can offset detrimental effects to teeth with oral delivery of fluoride by using fluoridated toothpaste daily.

If there is an excess in the diet:

- Preeruptively, it causes dental fluorosis which is manifested by intrinsic staining and appears as parchment white spots in its mildest form and dark brown porosities in its most severe form.
- Posteruptively, it has topical protective effects against dental caries and excess is excreted.

IRON

Iron is needed for the synthesis of hemoglobin. A deficiency in the diet can cause glossitis and dysphagia (difficulty swallowing). The papilla of the tongue becomes atrophied and give a shiny, smooth, red appearance. It causes mucous membranes to appear ashen gray, as with anemia; it also can cause the occurrence of angular cheilitis.

ZINC

Zinc is a mineral that helps with wound healing. A deficiency would cause a delay in wound healing and the epithelium of the tongue to thicken, which would decrease the sensation of taste.

Zinc wound healing

PROTEIN

Protein is known as the nutrient for building, repair, and maintenance. It generally functions to help with formation and repair of all tissues.

Protein building, repair, maintence of tissue

- Preeruptively, it assists with the formation of maxilla, mandible, and periodontal tissues, and forms the matrix for enamel and dentin.
- Posteruptively, it repairs all tissues and forms antibodies to help resist infection.

If there is a deficiency of protein in the diet:

- Preeruptively, it can slow the development of bone and tooth structure, which results in crowded and rotated teeth posteruptively. Crowded and rotated teeth lend themselves to increased caries susceptibility.
- Posteruptively, it can slow tissue healing and cause degeneration of periodontal connective tissues, including the periodontal ligament, bone, and cementum.

ENVIRONMENTAL INFLUENCE ON TOOTH DEVELOPMENT

Some environmental substances, when either ingested or inhaled during the preeruptive stages of tooth development, can have a future negative impact on caries resistance and aesthetics.

- Research conducted on school-aged children established a direct relationship between high blood levels of lead and high incidence of dental caries. Children in urban areas had higher lead content in enamel than those living in rural areas.
- Cotinine, a byproduct of nicotine, has a direct relationship with increased caries in children exposed to second-hand smoke. Also, smoking increases cavity causing bacteria; therefore, when parents who smoke kiss their children, they transfer the bacteria from their mouths to their children's

mouths. Read the American Dental Hygienists' Association (ADHA) 2007 press release for information on exposing children to second-hand smoke. http://www.adha.org/media/releases/01172007_smoke.htm.

- Tetracycline causes permanent intrinsic tooth staining if ingested during tooth development. Pediatricians have discouraged prescribing the medication to pregnant women and infants since 1970s, but the effects can still be seen in some older dental patients whose teeth were affected by the drug.
- High levels of naturally occuring fluoride in drinking water can cause unsightly dental fluorosis, a condition that manifests as permanently brown mottled enamel. Patients whose drinking water comes from wells should have the mineral content checked yearly to assure that the fluoride level is safe.

Putting This Into Practice

The last patient of the morning, a 35-year-old female, is new to your practice and presents for initial assessment. Her last dental visit was 6 years ago and she had a "deep cleaning" and a few fillings replaced at that time. Her chief complaint today is sore, bleeding gums.

Medical history is unremarkable.

Extraoral examination reveals the following:

- Angular chelitis
- Few facial moles
- Infected bilateral ear piercing
- Wearing of contacts

Intraoral examination reveals the following:

- Smooth, red tongue
- Amalgam tattoo buccal of no. 19
- Aphthous ulcer on labial near no. 25

Gingival examination reveals the following:

- Generalized marginal redness
- Heavy bleeding upon probing

(continued)

Dental examination reveals the following:

- Past and present dental caries
- Impacted third molars
- Maxillary and mandibular anterior crowding

Based on the initial assessment information, comment on probable:

1. Maternal nutrition during fetal development
2. Preeruptive nutrition
3. Posteruptive nutrition

WEB RESOURCES

American Dental Association—Tooth Eruption Charts
    http://www.ada.org/public/games/animation/interface.asp

Position on Fluoride http://www.ada.org/public/topics/fluoride/facts/fluoridation_facts.pdf

Cleft Palate Foundation—About Cleft Lip and Palate http://www.cleftline.org/aboutclp/

National Institute of Nutrition—The Effect of Diet on Dental Health
    http://www.nin.ca/public.html/Publications/NinReview/winter97.html

PBS—Folic Acid and Spina Bifida http://www.pbs.org/newshour/health/folic acid/

Wide Smiles—Cleft Lip and Palate Resource http://www.widesmiles.org/

SUGGESTED READING

Alvarez JO, Caceda J, Woolley TW, et al. A longitudinal study of dental caries in the primary teeth of children who suffered from infant malnutrition. *J Dent Res* 1993;72(12): 1573–1576.

Alvarez JO. Nutrition, tooth development, and dental caries. *J Coll Surg Edinb* 2001;46(6): 320–328.

Billings RJ, Berkowitz RJ, Watson G. Teeth. *Pediatrics* 2004;113(Suppl 4):1120–1127.

Browne D, Whelton H, O'Mullane D. Fluoride metabolism and fluorosis. *J Dent* 2005;33(3): 177–186.

Den Besten PK. Mechanism and timing of fluoride effects on developing enamel. *J Public Health Dent* 1999;59(4):247–252.

Do LG, Spencer AJ. Risk benefit balance in the use of fluoride among young children. *J Dent Res* 2007;86(8):723–728.

Gemmel A. Blood lead level and dental caries in school-aged children. *Environ Health perspect* 2002;110(10):A625–A630.

Moss M, Lanphear BP, Auinger P. Association of dental caries and blood lead levels. *JAMA* 1999;281:2294–2298.

Oliveira MJ, Paiva SM, Martins LH, et al. Fluoride intake by children at risk for the development of dental fluorosis: comparison of regular dentifrices and flavoured dentifrices for children. *Caries Res* 2007;41(6):460–466.

Osso D, Tinanoff N, Romberg E, et al. Relationship of naturally occurring fluoride in Carroll County, Maryland to aquifers, well depths, and fluoride supplementation prescribing behaviors. *J Dent Hyg* 2008;82(1):10.

Pizzo G, Piscopo MR, Pizzo I, et al. Community water fluoridation and caries prevention: a critical review. *Clin Oral Investig* 2007;11(3):189–193.

Robinson C, Connell S, Kirkham J, et al. The effect of fluoride on the developing tooth. *Caries Res* 2004;38(3):268–276.

SaRoriz Fonteles C, Zero DT, Moss ME, et al. Fluoride concentrations in enamel and dentin of primary teeth after pre- and postnatal fluoride exposure. *Caries Res* 2005;39(6):505–508.

Whelton HP, Ketley CE, McSweeney F, et al. A review of fluorosis in the European Union: prevalence, risk factors and aesthetic issues. *Community Dent Oral Epidemiol* 2004; 32(Suppl 1):9–18.

Yaffe S, Bierman W, Cann H, et al. Requiem for tetracyclines. *Pediatrics* 1975;55(1):142–143.

CHAPTER 14

DIETARY CONSIDERATIONS FOR THE LIFECYCLE

OBJECTIVES

Upon completion of this chapter, the reader will be able to:

1 Discuss the importance of balanced weight during pregnancy and the outcomes for either extreme: obesity or underweight

2 Define neural tube defects and identify the nutrient deficiency related to its occurrence

3 List the reasons for failure of an infant to thrive and explain how it affects physical, mental, and social growth

4 Explain television commercial influence on a child's diet

5 List good food choices for after-school snacks

6 Discuss the teenage culture and how it affects eating patterns.

7 Describe the differences in nutrient needs between males and females during the teenage years

8 Identify oral needs of the young and older adult due to physiologic changing

9 Discuss how healthy eating throughout the lifecycles can stave off chronic disease

KEY TERMS

Child	Older Adult	Prenatal
Failure to Thrive	Pica	Neural-Tube Defect
Gastroesophageal Reflux	Picky Eaters	Teenager
Disease (GERD)	Pregnancy Myths	Toddler
Lactose Intolerant	Premature	Young Adult

Good nutrition is vital for growth and health on the life continuum. Eating well for mother and child is important before pregnancy and continues to be important until death. Our bodies require the same basic nutrients our entire lives, but the recommended *quantities* for each vary as our physiologic needs change with aging.

General information on what to include in our diets to keep our bodies healthy for each stage of the lifecycle can be found in basic nutrition textbooks. This chapter includes highlights of those recommendations and how the diet relates to the oral cavity at a specific point in the growth continuum.

Stages of the lifecycle can be divided in many different ways depending on the topic being discussed. Sometimes level of education attained is the dividing factor—preschool, K-12, college. Sometimes it is by decade—1 to 10, 11 to 20, 21 to 30, and so on. For the purpose of this chapter, the following stages will be used to discuss oral changes and suggested food selections for optimal oral health:

- **Prenatal**—fetal
- **Infant**—birth to 12 months
- **Toddler**—1 to 4 years
- **Child**—5 to 12 years
- **Teenager**—13 to 19 years
- **Young adult**—20 to 50 years
- **Older adult**—51 years and older

PRENATAL

Ideally, a woman wishing to conceive should prepare her body by practicing good nutrition months before the actual conception. Unfortunately, many women are unaware of their pregnancy in the early months, and by then, tooth development is already underway. If a mother is overweight or underweight throughout pregnancy, it increases her chance of medical complications.[1] Aiming for optimal weight and health before conception, during pregnancy, and after delivery will give the child the greatest start in life.

- Obesity increases the mother's chance of developing life-threatening diseases for herself and her fetus. There is an increased incidence of hypertension, diabetes, preeclampsia, and prolonged delivery for the mother and congenital central nervous system malformations for the fetus. Obese mothers frequently have vitamin D deficiency, which means the child she delivers will be deficient in Vitamin D also.[2]
- A pregnant mother who is severely underweight during pregnancy can be anemic and experience early delivery of a low–birth-weight baby.[3]

There are three well-known "**pregnancy myths**" that, in spite of a body of scientific study refuting them, continue to exist.

1. Eating for two
2. You lose a tooth for each child
3. Pregnant women crave unusual foods

Although the mother is eating to nourish herself and her baby, the body requires only an extra 300 cal/d beginning in the fourth month until delivery. The pregnant woman should try not to waste those 300 calories on simple carbohydrates and should consider including the following:

- Extra protein for fetal tissue synthesis
- Calcium for bone mineralization
- Foods rich in all the B complex vitamins for increase in energy metabolism
- Fluids for the 25% increased need to support increase in maternal blood volume

Many people still believe that a mother can lose "one tooth per child" because the growing baby draws calcium from the mother's teeth. There has been no evidence to support this theory, although there is a correlation between motherhood and periodontal disease, due to stress.[4] If teeth are lost during pregnancy, it is usually due to decay and pain. If the mother has sufficient calcium in her diet, there will be enough calcium available for the growing fetus. Early in the pregnancy, hormones cause an increase in calcium absorption and storage in the mother's body. If calcium is deficient in the diet, it may be taken from the mother's bones, where it has been stored for rapid fetal bone growth during the third trimester, but not from the teeth.

Pregnancy creates an altered sense of taste and smell. A pregnant woman may find that she loses taste for foods she once relished and that other foods smell bad and are no longer desired. Because of the changes in these two senses, eating patterns may seem very different. It is estimated that somewhere between 75%

and 90% of pregnant women experience at least one food craving and 50% to 85% have at least one food aversion. Most food cravings are for something sweet, such as ice cream. As with nonpregnant women, these cravings have been linked with emotional needs or changes in hormones. Food for Thought 14-1 lists food categories that are most often craved.

🍎 FOOD FOR THOUGHT 14-1

TYPE OF FOOD CRAVED DURING PREGNANCY

Sweets: 40%
Salty: 33%
Spicy: 17%
Sour: 10%

Some pregnant women report symptoms of **pica**—a condition where a person will crave and eat nonnutritive substances like dirt and laundry detergent. It is usually an indication of iron or other mineral deficiency but is not contingent on pregnancy, as males and females of any age have been reported with this condition.

Foods rich in calcium, phosphorus, and vitamin D are important in the pregnant woman's diet for her baby's healthy tooth formation. Tooth development

TABLE 14-1 Tooth Development	
Tooth	**Time of Formation**
Primary incisors	4–5 mo *in utero*
Primary molars	5–6 mo *in utero*
Permanent central incisors	3–4 mo
Permanent lateral incisors	10–12 mo (3–4 mo mandible)
Permanent canine	4–5 mo
Permanent premolars	1.5–2.5 yr
Permanent first molars	At birth
Permanent second molars	2.5–3 yr

begins as early as the sixth week after conception, and calcification of the primary teeth begins at 4 months *in utero*. Formation (not calcification) of many of the permanent teeth has already started by the time the baby is born. Table 14-1 charts tooth development for primary and permanent dentition.

A woman planning on becoming pregnant should make sure there are plenty of folate-rich foods in her diet or take a supplement containing at least 400 µg of folic acid. Studies have shown that women with a folate deficiency during pregnancy have a greater chance of having a child with a **neural tube defect**.[5] Food for Thought 14-2 provides a list of neural-tube defects, and Food for Thought 14-3 provides a list of foods rich in folate.

🍎 FOOD FOR THOUGHT 14-2

NEURAL-TUBE DEFECTS

- Spina bifida: embryonic failure of fusion of one or more vertebral arches
- Malformation of the brain and skull
- Anencephaly: absence of bones of the cranial vault and cerebral and cerebellar hemispheres
- Encephalocele: gap in the skull with herniation of the brain

---

🍎 FOOD FOR THOUGHT 14-3

FOODS RICH IN FOLATE

Dark-green leafy vegetables
Citrus fruit and juices
Fortified cereal
Broccoli
Asparagus
Legumes
Beans
Peas
Nuts

Foods that can carry food-borne illnesses and should be avoided while pregnant are raw eggs, raw meat, soft cheeses, and unpasteurized juice. Some herbs can also be harmful to the fetus and should only be taken if prescribed by the doctor.

It takes about 40 weeks for a fetus to fully develop but about 10% of births are **premature** with the infant being born before the 37th week of gestation. Organs are not completely formed so the infant stays in a neonatal intensive care unit until it is determined that all organs are functioning properly. Breast feeding is preferred for preterm babies as it is higher in protein and rich in nutrients. Many premature infants will have delayed eruption patterns and teeth that erupt with enamel defects, but current research states more studies are needed.[6]

INFANT

Infancy is a time of tremendous growth—weight usually triples by the first birthday. There are two important facts to learn about this time period—intestinal absorption is inefficient and renal function is immature. With this in mind, infant nutrition must be specialized. Breast milk and infant formula both contain all the nutrients necessary for this time of rapid growth and should be provided exclusively for infants aged 4 to 6 months. Cow's milk has higher protein content than breast milk or formula and taxes the kidneys, which is why pediatricians do not recommended it until after the age of 1. Introduction of solid foods should be handled one at a time so that possible allergies can be identified. By the age of 1 year, the immature motor development allows the infant to attempt to feed him- or herself with a spoon or grab a cup, and the diet changes to include more variety.

Around the age of 6 months, the first primary teeth erupt into the oral cavity. Parents should be counseled on cleaning the newly erupted teeth with soft baby toothbrushes or cloths. Information should be given on the dangers of putting the infant to bed with a bottle propped in their mouth.Early Childhood Caries (ECC) is of epidemic proportions and can be prevented by feeding the baby before putting them to bed (see Chapter 9).

Failure to Thrive

Sometimes infants do not exhibit rapid growth expected in this stage of the lifecycle. When infants **fail to thrive**, their weight is not proportional to their height and they rank in the bottom third or below of standard growth charts. They appear much smaller than infants of same sex and age and their physical, mental, and social skills are underdeveloped. It is well known that when a mother withholds her affection and nurturing touch, her baby will fail to thrive. But many times, the cause of failure to thrive is multifactorial and combines medical, emotional, psychosocial, and nutritional issues.

Medical causes are many such as chromosome abnormalities, defective organs like heart and lung that affect oxygen flow throughout the body, thyroid or other hormone deficiency, brain damage, cerebral palsy, metabolic disorders, low birth weight, chronic infections, and parasites.

Nutritional-related causes can be nutrient malabsorption, poor eating habits, gastric reflux, and lack of digestive enzymes. New parents with low socioeconomic standards and low nutrition intelligence quotient (IQ) are in a high-risk group for having infants who fail to thrive. Reversing the process can be as simple as educating the parent about well-balanced meals with high nutrient value and counseling about creating a social environment that encourages good eating habits.[7,8]

TODDLER

Toddlers are moving from a fluid diet to one that consists of more solid foods. This is the time for parents to set a good example, because eating habits learned as a toddler can last a lifetime. Many toddlers become "**picky eaters**," due to decrease in appetite since rate of growth has dropped. Appetites will be erratic, but toddlers should not be forced to eat when they are not hungry as it can lead to childhood obesity. See Food for Thought 14-4.

🍎 FOOD FOR THOUGHT 14-4

According to a 2003 Center for Disease Control report, 10% of toddlers are overweight and studies have shown that overweight toddlers are more likely to be iron deficient. An iron deficiency can affect a child's ability to learn.

Food for Thought 14-5 lists pediatrician recommendations for total fat intake for toddlers.

🍎 FOOD FOR THOUGHT 14-5

High cholesterol levels have been noted in children as young as 2-year-old.
   Pediatricians recommend that fat intake be kept around 30% of total daily calorie intake up to the age of 5 years.

🍎 FOOD FOR THOUGHT 14-6

Protein Energy Malnutrition (PEM) is the leading cause of childhood mortality in developing countries. It develops after weaning when the child's diet does not have enough protein to meet requirements for growth. A child with kwashiorkor, a form of PEM, will have thin arms and legs and large belly that is distended from edema.

It is not uncommon for toddlers to request the same foods for lunch and dinner in the same day, or for 5 days in a row. Because their calorie requirement has decreased, it is important for parents to guide their food choices to get the most nutrients from food. Snacking is an important part of the diet at this stage, so it is important to provide nutritious snack food versus snacks detrimental to teeth, such as fermentable carbohydrates.

Children have a tendency to model their eating patterns after parents. If fast food is a staple in the family diet, now is the time to teach children to make healthier food choices. Thirty percent of all children report eating fast foods on any given day.[9] Milk or water instead of soda, and a salad instead of french fries will go a long way in fostering healthy eating habits in other lifecycle stages. Food for Thought 14-7 lists healthy snack choices for toddlers. Eye-hand coordination is improving, and toddlers want to feed themselves. Mealtime can be messy but it is important to let the child develop the movements necessary for independent feeding.

🍎 FOOD FOR THOUGHT 14-7

HEALTHY SNACK SUGGESTIONS

- Sliced apples, pears, peaches, and grapes
- Slivers of carrots or celery with dip
- Bagels topped with peanut butter, smashed fruit, or cream cheese
- Soft taco rolls filled with leftover meat
- Cheese strips or cubes
- Yogurt
- Small crustless sandwiches
- Popcorn
- Peanut butter or cheese on crackers
- English muffin pizzas
- Tortillas with bean dip

SCHOOL-AGE CHILD

The period when children are in school continues the time when they form a lifelong relationship with food. Although the brain is the same size as an adult, the liver—where glucose is stored—is only about half as big. To maintain a steady blood glucose level, children need to eat more frequently—about every 4 hours. When children are not able to eat, their brains are depleted of glucose, which makes concentration in school difficult.

Food takes on social, emotional, and psychological implications. Preference for comfort foods can last a lifetime, and other food choices may take on reward significance. Rewarding a child with sweets can be a hard habit to break later in life. Food for Thought 14-8 asks questions that help determine the social, emotional, and psychological implications of food.

🍎 FOOD FOR THOUGHT 14-8

SOCIAL, EMOTIONAL, AND PSYCHOLOGICAL IMPLICATIONS OF FOOD

- When you think of being sick, do you think of a specific food?
- When you feel happy and successful, do you reach for a certain food?
- What foods remind you of being with friends?
- What is your all-time favorite food?
- When you feel sad, do you reach for a particular food?

The appetite of school-age child is usually very good, with snacks making up the majority of the daily calories. Snacks provide the child with calories needed to maintain high energy levels. At this stage, children enjoy most foods, but as one can imagine, vegetables are last choice. Children can be ravenous after school and head toward the refrigerator as soon as they return home. Stocking up on ready-to-eat healthy snacks can be a quick fix for their hunger. Many snacks are bought from fast food restaurants and vending machines, but these food choices are high in fat, sugar, and salt and low in fiber. If the majority of a child's daily calories are from these types of snacks, their bodies will become deficient in major nutrients. Studies show that the low-nutrient food selections at fast food restaurants and vending machines contribute to childhood obesity.[10] Parents should discourage day-long grazing and beverage sipping and set regular times for family meals to reduce both the caries potential of the diet and excess caloric intake. Vitamin/mineral supplements are very important as a back-up to an inadequate diet.

Females begin to require more iron as menstruation begins. This is also a time when they become aware of their body image. Parents should use caution with their own projection of body image, because this can influence how a growing young woman feels about her own body.

Children's eating patterns are greatly influenced by watching television. According to AC Nielsen Co, the average person watches 4 hours of television per day and 66% of American families watch television as they eat dinner. For a child, this factors out to 20,000—30-second TV commercials per year. When a child who is already obese views a food advertisement on TV, their food intake is increased by at least 100%.[11] If parents are at all concerned about their child keeping a healthy weight, they should monitor hours spent in front of the television and make sure it is off at mealtime.

For good oral health, an increase in calcium is needed at this age. There is exfoliation of primary teeth, eruption of permanent teeth, and a growth spurt in long bones. A diet rich in calcium, phosphorus, and vitamin D should be continued for healthy development of bones and teeth.

TEENAGERS

Teenagers have the worst diets of any age-group. Their diets are influenced by everyone and everything, except their parents: peer pressure, acne control, weight control, and muscle building. The teenage years are a period of very rapid physical growth, second only to infancy, and of intense stress and change. Hormonal changes affect every body organ, including the brain. About half of adult bone structure is deposited during adolescence and continues another 10 years. Nutrient and energy needs are greatly accelerated.

More responsibility is added to teenagers' lives as they obtain driver's licenses, begin dating, and work part-time jobs. Their busy lifestyles can dictate when, where, and what they eat. Unfortunately, their food selection usually does not meet their increased energy needs. Teenagers' favorite foods have been identified as hamburgers, pizza, fried chicken, Tex-Mex, french fries, spaghetti, ice cream, orange juice, and soda. Sodas replace milk and fruit juice, which causes inadequate calcium intake. Teenagers drink twice as much soda as milk, whereas the opposite was true 20 years ago. The average male drinks two cans per day and the female slightly less. That amounts to more than 868 cans of soda per teenager each year, with a price tag of $54 billion yearly.

This is also an age when nutrient requirements differ for males and females. Females have reached their maximum linear growth and begin to increase their percentage of body fat. This is also the time when they should be storing calcium

TABLE 14-2   Growth and Nutrient Needs for Males and Females

Males	Females
Maximum linear growth is reached by age 15	Maximum linear growth is reached by age 13
Eat twice as much as females of same age	Interested in achieving a slender figure through calorie reduction
2,500 calories for ages 11–14	2,200 calories for ages 11–18
3,000 calories for ages 15–18	Need more iron because of monthly blood loss

for peak bone mass and to stave off osteoporosis in later years. Males, on the other hand, are building up to their maximum linear growth and begin to develop more bone and muscle mass. A 15-year-old male can consume 4,000 cal/d just to maintain his current weight. More calories should be added for the extra energy needs. Table 14-2 compares the difference in growth and nutrient needs between males and females.

Both genders place tremendous importance on body shape and image during the teenage years. Females may worry they are not thin enough and males may worry they are not as muscular as they should be. The roots of many eating disorders begin at this stage, and if allowed to progress can be a lifelong battle to remain mentally and physically healthy (see Chapter 15). Tooth bleaching/whitening and sporting grills are important to this age-group as they explore ways to express their self-image. Visit the ADA website to learn more about their stance on grills. http://www.ada.org/public/topics/grills.asp and policy on effectiveness of tooth whitening products. http://www.ada.org/prof/resources/positions/statements/whiten2.asp.

Peer pressure during the teenage years can be intense. Behaviors that may seem hip, trendy, and the norm for the peer group can lead to regret in later life. Smoking and drug abuse are the two, which are of dental concern with 35% of high school students reporting some use of tobacco[12] and 2.3 million 12 to 17 year olds abuse of at least one controlled prescription drug. Developing an addiction to tobacco or drugs can be hard to shake and if continued into adulthood will cause detrimental oral changes. Research has established a direct cause and effect relationship between smoking, poor oral health, and malnutrition with periodontal disease and dental caries. The sooner abuse is identified, the better the chance of successful intervention. The American

Dental Association has developed policies for dental health care workers to recognize the signs of abuse and their role in managing the issue. Visit The 2005 ADA House of Delegates adopted policy on guidelines related to alcohol, nicotine, and/or drug use by child or adolescent patients for a complete report. http://www.ada.org/prof/resources/pubs/adanews/adanewsarticle.asp?articleid=2341

Consider the following factors for teenage diet influence:

- Rate of very rapid growth
- Eat a typically unhealthy diet
- Nutrient needs for males and females differ
  - Females need more calcium and iron
  - Males have an increase in all major nutrient needs
- Food choices are influenced by peers
- Heightened awareness of body shape

YOUNG ADULTHOOD

Twenty-first century adults are very busy people. Lunch is usually eaten away from home, many meals are skipped, and dinner is prepared as quickly as possible. It is a time of multiple stresses and multitasking: raising children, managing a home, and keeping track of both household and work schedules. In spite of all this "busyness," nutrient needs are reduced. There is a gradual slowing of metabolic rate that goes unnoticed at first, but emerges to consciousness somewhere around the age of 50. Adults will notice that they may eat less and still gain weight. Organ function begins to become less efficient around the age of 30 and continues to decline as we age. Just as you notice subtle changes in texture, color, and amount of hair as well as a "loosening" of the skin, internal organs are also going through gentle changes in function. All senses begin to diminish. Ability to see and hear slowly fades and can make reading labels and recipes difficult. Inability to taste well may lead to overseasoning. The thirst mechanism begins to fail, which can cause dehydration.

Evidence of chronic diseases may start to manifest—diabetes, cardiovascular disease, and hypertension to name a few. After years of improper nutrition or perhaps bad genes, young adults can no longer say "It won't happen to me". The average age of Diabetes II diagnosis is late 40s, and 30 to 50 years for hypertension. According to the American Heart Association Heart Disease and Stroke Statistics, one out of every three adults has one or more types of cardiovascular disease. (http://www.americanheart.org/downloadable/heart/1200078608862HS_Stats%202008.final .pdf).

Many adults will complain of other digestive irregularities such as lactose intolerance and gastric reflux disease. Both disorders can take away the pleasure of eating and limit choices in food.

- **Lactose intolerant** means that small intestines no longer produce the enzyme lactase that breaks apart lactose in dairy products. If the small intestines do not deal with the lactose, it passes on to the colon where bacteria metabolize it and produce gas. For some, it is part of the natural aging process when our diets no longer contain dairy as a main source of nutrition. Someone who is lactose intolerant will experience diarrhea, bloating, gas, or nausea anywhere from 30 minutes to 2 hours after eating some form of dairy product.
- **Gastroesophageal reflux disease** (GERD) occurs when digested food/bile is allowed to backwash into the esophagus, because of malfunctioning sphincter between the lower esophagus and upper portion of the stomach. The acidic contents irritate the lining of the esophagus causing significant burning sensation. If left untreated, it can potentially cause narrowing of the esophagus, ulcerous sores, or cancer. People who smoke, are obese, pregnant, have a hiatal hernia, or medical condition that causes the stomach to empty slower (Diabetes) are prone to GERD. Prescriptions and over-the-counter medications can offer some relief, and weight control and eating smaller meals reduce number of episodes. Foods that can worsen the condition are alcohol, chocolate, fatty fried, citrus, garlic, onions, mint, tomatoes, and anything spicy.

Consider the following factors for teenage diet influence:

- Metabolic rate slows.
- Organ function begins to diminish.
- Sight and hearing are impaired.
- Taste sensation is reduced.
- There is an inability to sense thirst.
- There is an overall reduced enjoyment of food.

Oral changes parallel overall body changes. If proper oral hygiene has not been a routine practice, devastation from periodontal disease and dental caries is present: bone loss, multiple missing, and/or restored teeth. Xerostomia becomes a concern as the aging process causes mucosa to be less lubricated, thirst mechanism diminishes, and practicing polypharmacy is common. Dry mouth equals poor saliva, which can equal dental caries in enamel and on roots exposed from recession. Adult patients should be reminded of the importance of thorough daily oral hygiene, including foods that stimulate saliva, and the use of home fluoride for sensitive and exposed root surfaces.

OLDER ADULT

With the state of our current medical technology, life expectancy has increased and some people live into their 100s. Studies are ongoing about the calorie-reduction diet and its relationship to longevity.[13] The elderly age-group is different from those previously mentioned in that biologic age varies widely with chronological age. A person who has reached the age of 70 could have a biologic age of a 50-year-old, and *vice versa*. Depending on genetics, life experiences, and ability to resist disease, our bodies age at different rates. Good nutrition plays an important role in keeping the body free from disease and the dentition healthy. From the age of 50, calorie intake should decrease and physical activity should increase. Lean body mass declines (as a result of decrease in protein intake) and adipose tissue increases.

Many elderly patients will report polypharmacy—taking multiple medications, most of which cause salivary gland hypofunction (xerostomia). Eating with a very dry mouth becomes uncomfortable. Foods will stick to teeth and soft tissues, allowing spicy foods to burn unlubricated mucosa. Each bolus of food might seem to "stick" going down. This can lead to eliminating dry, sticky, and crunchy foods and adding soft, bland items to the diet.

With a higher incidence of root caries and periodontal disease at this stage, good nutrition is very important to maintain a healthy dentition. Loss of teeth makes chewing difficult, and the elimination of crunchy foods with meals minimizes the flow of good saliva. Teeth do not get the good buffering effects of sodium bicarbonate, calcium, and phosphorus. Those who suffer from tooth loss or wear dentures do not have the powerful grinding force of a natural dentition and may prefer a bland soft diet to one that includes crunchy fibrous foods. The following list includes some common reasons for poor eating habits of the elderly:

- Dysphagia: swallowing problems
- Altered gastrointestinal (GI) motility: constipation lining of intestinal tract is not replaced as often
- Economic: fixed incomes mean a greater percentage of the elderly at poverty level, with failing health and high medical bills
- Psychological: apathy and depression cause decreased appetite and interest in food
- Side effects of medication and social factors (inability to drive and living alone); most of their friends may have passed on
- Eating meals out frequently: meet in groups at fast food restaurants for socialization and to take advantage of senior discounts

COUNSELING PATIENTS

Pregnancy
- Prenatal vitamins are a good idea, even if just considering a pregnancy.
- Do not eat twice as much just because you are "eating for two." Around the fourth month of pregnancy, increase daily calorie intake by 300 but include extra protein, calcium, and food rich in vitamins and minerals in those extra calories.
- Get at least 400 µg of folate in your diet or supplement to prevent neural-tube defects.
- Increase fluid intake.
- Avoid caffeine, alcohol, tobacco, and any drug not prescribed by your physician. All pass through the placental barrier and affect the growing child.
- Minimize processed foods from the diet because all have artificial colorants and flavoring, and it is not well known how these affect the growing child.
- Take adequate iron to avoid iron-deficiency anemia.
- Adequate calcium, phosphorus, and vitamin D intake ensures good calcification of your child's teeth.

Infancy
- If formula is made with distilled or bottled water that does not contain fluoride, ask the pediatrician if fluoride supplementation is needed.
- Primary teeth are beginning to erupt into the oral cavity. Prevent ECC by not putting the infant to bed with a bottle. Fluid pools around teeth, causing dental caries.
- Use water to quench thirst and juice occasionally because of acidic pH that contributes to ECC.
- The crowns of permanent teeth are in a stage of calcification, so adequate calcium, phosphorus, and Vitamin D are required.

Toddlers
- Have suggestions for healthy snacks readily available when counseling.
- Consider level of income and availability of foods.

School-Age Child
- Avoid using food as punishment, reward, or consolation.
- There is a tendency for the school-age child to choose soda over milk, but this practice should be discouraged.
- Involve children in meal preparation; they are more apt to eat what they cook.

Teenagers
- Appeal to their body image, such as muscular development.
- Praise good food choices and ignore the others.
- Encourage healthy snacks—cooked meats, nuts, cheese, milk, fruit, peanut butter, and popcorn.
- This is the time when young women should begin acquiring a surplus of calcium in their bones. Counsel as to how to incorporate more calcium in the diet.

Young Adult
- Between 30 and 40, resorption of existing bone begins to exceed formation of new bone, resulting in a net loss of bone.
- Bone growth and shaping of the growing skeleton cease at maturity, and remodeling takes over.
- Bone loss happens in both males and females, and once it begins, it continues throughout the rest of life.
- Osteoporosis is the result of excessive bone loss.

Older Adult
- The greatest reduction in nutrient and energy needs is in the elderly years.
- Increase fiber intake.
- Decrease fat intake.
- Recommend a senior vitamin/mineral supplement.
- Ensure adequate calcium intake to avoid osteoporosis.
- Multiple medications can alter how the body absorbs vitamins and minerals.
- There is an increased need for exercise, which will resist bone resorption for prevention of osteoporosis.
- The elderly may restrict fluid intake due to incontinence or nocturia.

Putting This Into Practice

1. Obtain an informational brochure on the nutrient content of foods served at two of your favorite fast-food restaurants.
   a. Compare the fat, cholesterol, carbohydrates, and sodium for your favorite selections at each restaurant.
   b. Is one choice better than the other?

(continued)

c. How could you boost the nutrient content of your selection and at the same time reduce fat and sodium?

d. What would you suggest to improve the selections of a client who frequents fast-food restaurants?

NAME OF RESTAURANT

Nutrient	First Selection	Second Selection
Saturated fat		
Total fat		
Cholesterol		
Carbohydrate		
Sodium		

2. If your client asked your opinion on what to provide as an after-school snack for their school-age child, what suggestions would you give them?

3. Give an example of a healthy snack for each of the following age-groups:
   a. Toddler
   b. School-age child
   c. Teenager
   d. Adult
   e. Elderly

WEB RESOURCES

Academy of General Dentistry—Children's Nutrition: What Foods Cause Tooth Decay in Children? http://www.agd.org/consumer/topics/childrensnutrition/main.html

Academy of General Dentistry—Development Chart for Feeding Infants
http://www.agd.org/consumer/topics/childrensnutrition/weaningchart.html

American Dental Association—Good Oral Health Begins in the Womb
http://www.ada.org/public/media/releases/0202_release06.asp

Better Food Choices at Fast-Food Restaurants (from the Minnesota Attorney General)
http://www.olen.com/food/book.html

Calorie Content of Fast Food http://www.diet-i.com/calorie_chart/fast-food.htm

Economic Research Service—Nutrient-to-Calorie Density
   http://www.ers.usda.gov/briefing/DietAndHealth/data/nutrients/table8.htm

Fast Food Finder by Olen Publishing http://www.olen.com/food/index.html

Fast Food Nutrition Fact Explorer http://www.fatcalories.com/

Ingredient List and Nutritional Counts of Select Restaurants
   http://www.dietriot.com/fff/rest.html

Living Longer: A History of Longevity http://www.pbs.org/stealingtime/living/history.htm

REFERENCES

1. Sahu MT, Agarwal A, Das V, et al. Impact of maternal body mass index on obstetric outcome. *J Obstet Gynaecol Res* 2007;33(5):655–659.
2. Bodnar LM, Catov JM, Roberts JM, et al. Prepregnancy obesity predicts poor vitamin D status in mothers and their neonates. *J Nutr* 2007;137(11):2437–2442.
3. Sebire NJ, Jolly M, Harris J, et al. Is maternal underweight really a risk factor for adverse pregnancy outcome? A population-based study in London. *BJOG* (2001);108(1):61–66.
4. Scheutz F, Baelum V, Matee MI, et al. Motherhood and dental disease. *Community Dent Health* 2002;19(2):67–72.
5. Centers for Disease Control and Prevention. Use of supplements containing folic acid among women of childbearing age—United States. *MMWR Morb Mortal Wkly Rep* 2008;57(1):5–8.
6. Paulsson L, Bondemark L, Söderfeldt BA. Systematic review of the consequences of premature birth on palatal morphology, dental occlusion, tooth-crown dimensions, and tooth maturity and eruption. *Angle Orthod* 2004;74(2):269–279.
7. Olsen EM. Failure to thrive still a problem definition. *Clin Pediatr* 2006;45(1):1–6.
8. Block RW, Krebs NF. Failure to thrive as a manifestation of child neglect. *Pediatrics* 2005;116(5):1234–1237.
9. Bowman SA, Gortmaker SL, Ebbeling CB, et al. Effects of fast-food consumption on energy intake and diet quality among children in a national household survey. *Pediatrics* 2004;113(1):112–118.
10. Hurley J, Liebman B. Kid's cuisine. What would you like with your fries? *Nutr Action Health Lett* 2004:12–15.
11. University of Liverpool 2007. April 25, *TV Food advertisements increase obese children's appetite by 134%*. Science Daily.
12. Tomar SL. Dentistry's role in tobacco control. *J Am Dent* 2001;132(Suppl 30–35):30S–35S.
13. Johnson JB, Laub DR, John S. The effect on health of alternate day calorie restriction: eating less and more than needed on alternate days prolongs life. *Med Hypotheses* 2006;67(2):209–211.

SUGGESTED READING

Allen RE, Myers AL. Nutrition in toddlers. *Am Fam Physician* 2006;74(9):1527–1532.

Alm A, Fahraeus C, Wendt LK, et al. Body adiposity status in teenagers and snacking habits in early childhood in relation to approximal caries at 15 years of age. *Int J Paediatr Dent* 2008;18(3):189–196.

Berkey CS, Rockett HR, Gillman MW, et al. Longitudinal study of skipping breakfast and weight change in adolescents. *Int J Obes Relat Metab Disord* 2003;27(10):1258–1266.

Brotanek JM, Gosz J, Weitzman M, et al. Iron deficiency in early childhood in the United States: risk factors and racial/ethnic disparities. *Pediatrics* 2007;120(3):568–575.

Chen C. Adolescent diets and oral health. *Probe* 2004;38(1):16–20.

Collins K. *Help for parents of picky eaters. MSNBC News*, July 18, 2004.

Connor SM. Food related advertising on preschool television: building brand recognition in young viewers. *Pediatrics* 2006;118(4):1478–1485.

Drewett RF, Corbett SS, Wright CM. Physical and emotional development, appetite and body image in adolescents who failed to thrive as infants. *J Child Psychol Psychiatry* 2006; 47(5):524–531.

Feldman R, Keren M, Gross-Rozval O, et al. Mother-child touch patterns in infant feeding disorders: relation to maternal, child, and environmental factors. *J Am Acad Child Adolesc Pshyciatry* 2004;43(9):1089–1097.

Fitzsimons D, Dwyer JT, Palmer C, et al. Nutrition and oral health guidelines for pregnant women, infants, and children. *J Am Diet Assoc* 1998;98(3):264.

Guelinckx I, Devlieger R, Beckers K, et al. Maternal obesity: pregnancy complications, gestational weight gain and nutrition. *Obes Rev* 2008;9(2):140–150.

He Q. BMI monitoring in the management of obesity in toddlers. *Am Fam Physician*. 2006; 74(9):1483–1484.

Lustig RH. The 'skinny' on childhood obesity: how our western environment starves kids' brains. *Pediatr Ann* 2006;35(12):898–902, 905–907.

Marshall TA, Warren JJ, Hand JS, et al. Oral health, nutrient intake and dietary quality in the very old. *J Am Dent Assoc* 2002;133(10):1369–1379.

Paeratakul S, Ferdinand DP, Champagne CM, et al. Fast-food consumption among US adults and children: dietary and nutrient intake profile. *J Am Diet Assoc* 2003;103(19): 1296–1297.

Percy MS. Oral health of adolescents–its more than dental caries. *MCN Am J Matern Child Nurs* 2008;33(1):26–31.

Psoter W, Gebrian B, Prophete S, et al. Effect of early childhood malnutrition on tooth eruption in Haitian adolescents. *Community Dent Oral Epidemiol* 2008;36(2):179–189.

Robin L. Healthy eating is essential for healthy teeth in young children. *Probe* 2004;38(1): 14–15.

Ryan-Harshman M, Aldoori W. Folic acid and prevention of neural-tube defects. *Can Fam Physician* 2008;54(1):36–38.

Sahyoun NR, Lin CL, Krall E. Nutritional status of the older adult is associated with dentition status. *J Am Diet Assoc* 2003;103(1):61–66.

Vandewater EA, Shim MS, Caplovitz AG. Linking obesity and activity level with children's television and video game use. *J Adolesc* 2004;27(1):71–85.

Vargas CM, Dye BA, Hayes KL. Oral health status of older rural adults in the United States. *J Am Dent Assoc* 2003;134(4):479–486.

PART VI

NUTRITIONAL COUNSELING

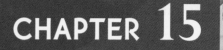

EATING DISORDERS

OBJECTIVES

Upon completion of this chapter, the reader will be able to:

1 Cite statistics for those affected with eating disorders

2 Explain the difference between anorexia nervosa and bulimia nervosa.

3 Describe the psychology behind binge eating

4 Outline home care advice for individuals with eating disorders

5 Identify physical and oral signs of eating disorders

6 Explain the etiology of eating disorders

7 Help develop a comprehensive dental treatment plan for individuals with eating disorders

8 Use good communication techniques when treating individuals with eating disorders

9 List four other less common eating disorders

KEY TERMS

Ana	Bulimics	Mia
Anorexia Athletica	Compulsive Overeating	Orthorexia Nervosa
Anorexia Nervosa	Eating Disorders	Pica
Binge	Emotional Triggers	Purging
Body Dysmorphic Disorder	Lanugo	

Eating disorders are listed as "mental disorders" by the National Institute of Mental Health. For an individual with an eating disorder, the thought process malfunctions and instead of viewing food as something good and life sustaining, it becomes the enemy and is either severely restricted or gorged upon as self-punishment. The figures of those afflicted are staggering: 70 million worldwide and 24 million in the United States. Ninety percent of those afflicted are young and females in the age-group of 15 and 24 and the other 10% are males and either very young or old. It has become a global epidemic and success of treatment hinges on bringing the deep dark secret into the open, to see it for what it is, and that can be a very emotionally painful process.

Treatment includes medicating with antidepressants and psychiatric and nutritional counseling. Earlier the treatment begins, the greater the success. Controlling food intake may be the only sense of control a person with an eating disorder may feel in their lives. It signifies self-discipline and achievement and they will not give it up easily. Unfortunately, about 20% of those affected by eating disorders will succumb to death, making it the highest mortality rate for a mental illness.

Etiology is multifactorial and influenced by social, psychological, and biologic factors. Each disorder may have distinct physical symptoms with oral manifestations, and it is the oral complications that eventually lead the patient with an eating disorder to the dental office. Since the dental auxiliary is the person most likely to take the medical/dental history and provide the first oral examination, he or she may also be the first to identify the disease. Dental auxiliaries usually are not regarded as people of authority or as threatening to the patient, and because of this, they may be the perfect choice for a confidant. Counseling and treatment for the specific eating disorder is not among the dental professional's responsibilities, but restoring oral problems and prevention of oral complications caused by the disease are both necessary and expected.

There are three main eating disorders:

- Anorexia nervosa—**Ana** for short
- Bulimia nervosa—**Mia** for short
- Binge eating

ETIOLOGY OF EATING DISORDERS

Eating disorders are not contagious like a cold or flu. They develop from deep emotional disturbances that manifest as extreme attitudes toward food. **Emotional triggers** can be psychological or social/interpersonal: fear of getting fat as a body goes through puberty, loss of control, ill-defined sense of self, distorted body image, stress, and anxiety. Most individuals with eating disorders exhibit combined mental disorders and will also suffer with depression and anxiety. Occasionally, there will be a biological factor contributing to an eating disorder such as reduced seratonin levels in the brain or reduced number of fungiform papillae on the tongue.[1]

[handwritten: depression + anxiety]

Psychological Factors

- Low self-esteem and shame
- Feelings of inadequacy or lack of control in life
- Depression, anxiety, anger, and loneliness

Social/Interpersonal Factors

- Media pressure that misrepresents perfectly thin bodies as being preferable
- Nonacceptance of beauty in diversity (narrow views)
- Difficulty with family and interpersonal relationships
- Difficulty in expressing emotions and feelings
- History of being teased about weight
- History of sexual abuse

Media plays a huge role in propagating eating disorders by employing unnaturally thin models and insinuating that all should aspire to look like them. Young females are especially prone to influence, getting "thinspiration" from fashion magazines. With the recent death of a Brazilian model because of anorexia, many designers are refusing to employ waif-like models, which may or may not reverse the trend. Only time will tell. The following are facts referenced on the website of National Eating Disorders Association (NEDA):

- Eighty percent of American women are dissatisfied with their appearance.
- The average American woman is 5 ft 4 in. tall and weighs 140 lb. Compare that to the average American model, who is 5 ft 11 in. tall and weighs 117 lb.
- Most fashion models are thinner than 98% of American women.
- Eighty-one percent of 10-year-olds are afraid of being fat.
- Fifty-one percent of 9- and 10-year-olds feel better about themselves if they are on a diet.
- Ninety-one percent of women on college campuses attempt to control their weight through dieting.

[handwritten: 80% of women are dissatisfied w/ appearance]

- Ninety-five percent of all dieters will regain their lost weight in 1 to 5 years.
- Forty billion dollars is spent on dieting and diet-related products each year.

BIOLOGIC FACTORS

- Unbalanced brain chemicals that signal and control hunger and satiety
- Genetic predisposition
- Unbalanced hormones
- Reduced serotonin levels in the brain
- Reduced numbers of fungiform papillae

🍎 FOOD FOR THOUGHT 15-1

If you know a friend of relative with an eating disorder, be honest and tell them of your concern in a loving and supportive way. Let them know of your suspicions and worry for them early on. Do not wait until the disease has wreaked havoc physically, mentally, and dentally. If they would not admit it, do not push. Just let them know you are there if they need you.

ANOREXIA NERVOSA

Anorexia nervosa literally means nervous lack of appetite. It is mainly a disease that develops in young females shortly after puberty or during adolescence when the body begins to change. Its characteristic self-imposed weight loss stems from a distorted attitude toward eating and body weight. Anorexics appear painfully thin, yet even though they look like skin on a skeleton, in their minds they still look fat. They look in a mirror and see pockets of fat where there are none. Food is the enemy, and every minute of every day the anorexic is thinking of ways to lose weight. Individuals with anorexia nervosa will severely restrict food or use punitive exercise sessions to burn any calories consumed.[2] They are brilliant when it comes to knowing calorie content of food, calculating total calories consumed, and how many hours of exercise it will take to burn what they have eaten. This self-imposed starvation wreaks havoc on the body, and if left untreated, an electrolyte imbalance can cause cardiac arrest and, ultimately, death. Figure 15-1 lists some of the symptoms of anorexia nervosa.

Most anorexics are very secretive and will exhibit behaviors to conceal their starvation tactics: denial that there is a problem, wearing clothing that makes them

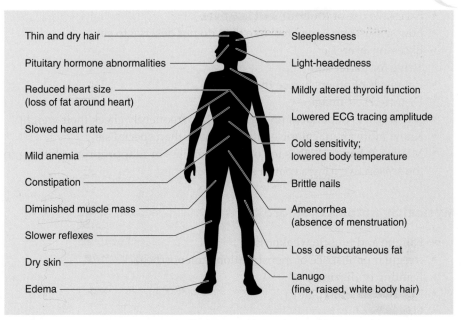

Thin and dry hair

Pituitary hormone abnormalities

Reduced heart size
(loss of fat around heart)

Slowed heart rate

Mild anemia

Constipation

Diminished muscle mass

Slower reflexes

Dry skin

Edema

Sleeplessness

Light-headedness

Mildly altered thyroid function

Lowered ECG tracing amplitude

Cold sensitivity;
lowered body temperature

Brittle nails

Amenorrhea
(absence of menstruation)

Loss of subcutaneous fat

Lanugo
(fine, raised, white body hair)

FIGURE 15-1   **Symptoms of anorexia nervosa. ECG, electrocardiogram.**

appear of normal weight, lying about eating habits, avoidance of being weighed or putting rocks or other heavy items in their pockets before stepping on a scale.

Proanorexic websites exist to support anorexics in food restriction efforts, thus preventing them from talking about their disorder with family and professionals who can actually help.[3] Visit www.community.livejournal.com/proanorexia to read livetime comments of anorexics and bulimics.

🍎 FOOD FOR THOUGHT 15-2

For a glimpse into the mind of an anorexic or bulimic, Google pro ana for a list of websites created by individuals with and for eating disorders. You will find blogs, recipes, pictures, you tube videos, and a lot of other information in support of eating disorders.

Signs and Symptoms

- Terrified of gaining weight
- Excuses for not eating meals
- Cook for others but then they do not eat themselves

- Excessive use of diuretics and laxatives
- Low self-esteem—may feel like they do not deserve to eat
- Excessive exercise
- Strive for perfection
- Put needs of others before their own
- Distorted self-image
- Self-worth is dependent on weight—they frequently check their weight
- Know more about caloric content of foods than specialists
- May wear baggy clothes to cover up thinness or inappropriate clothing for the season (wearing a coat in summer)

Physical Symptoms of Anorexia

- Fatigue and muscle weakness
- Irregular or absence of menstruation (amenorrhea)
- Fainting or dizziness
- Pale complexion (pallor)
- Headaches
- Irregular heartbeats
- Cold hands and feet
- Loss of bone mass
- Electrolyte imbalance
- Insomnia
- Low potassium—cardiac arrest

Oral Signs of Anorexia

- Anemic tissues
- Chapped lips

You may notice the following physical symptoms in a person with anorexia nervosa when the person is in the treatment chair:

- Painfully thin
- May have appearance of **lanugo**—a light fuzzy hair on face
- Avoids eye contact
- Dehydration
- Dry brittle skin and nails
- Low blood pressure, lowered metabolic rate, and always cold

BULIMIA NERVOSA

Bulimics are usually of average weight. The classic symptom of this disease is binging on food and then purging. A diagnosis is made if binging/purging occurs at least twice a week for at least 3 months. It is a cycle of overeating, feeling guilty about overeating, purging, and then feeling relief. Figure 15-2 illustrates the cycle of binging and purging.

The amount of food used to **binge** can vary according to the perception of the person who suffers from this disorder. For some, eating one cookie may be binging, and for others, it may be eating two whole packages of cookies, a whole pizza, and a half-gallon of ice cream in one sitting. **Purging** is not only vomiting, but can also be use of laxatives and/or enemas, excessive exercising, fasting, and use of diuretics and/or diet pills. Vomiting with the help of the first two fingers down the throat is the most reported means of purging. Many times, a callous will develop on the fingers used to help purge as (not because) they rub against the central incisors. Most bulimics are women and the disease is not checked by culture and nationality as it has made its way into homes around the world.[4] Bulimia is common in baby-boomer females aged 35 years and older who are struggling with the pressures of a career, aging, and the narrow view of the media-hyped symbol of beauty. The disease crosses generations as children learn from mothers who struggle with self-image issues, and there is a very high incidence of bulimia among college students.

Some precipitants of binging episodes include anxiety, stress, threat of physical harm, disruption in relationships, boredom, and societal pressure.

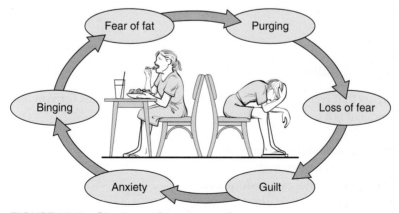

FIGURE 15-2 Binging and purging cycle.

[Handwritten margin notes: bulimics are usual weight; 2x/wk; 3 mo. Purging vomiting use of laxatives]

Signs and Symptoms of Bulimia

- Binge eating
- Visits bathroom immediately after eating
- Vomiting
- Misuse of laxatives and diuretics
- Use of diet pills
- Fasting
- Depression
- Excessive exercising
- Avoids restaurants and planned social meals

Physical Signs of Bulimia

- Broken blood vessels in eyes
- Fatigue
- Muscle weakness
- Irregular heartbeats
- Dizziness
- Headaches
- Dehydration
- Amenorrhea
- Electrolyte imbalance and low blood pressure
- Chest pains
- Stomach ulcers
- Edema in hands and feet
- Cardiac arrest
- Death

Oral Signs of Bulimia

Gastric acids that pass through the oral cavity can leave clues for you, indicating that your client is a bulimic.

- Enamel erosion/brittle enamel
- Dentinal hypersensitivity
- Extrusion of amalgam restorations
- Xerostomia
- Swollen parotid glands
- Erythematous oral tissues and red palate

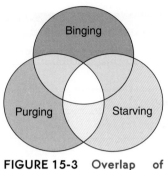

FIGURE 15-3 Overlap of eating disorders.

- Chronic sore throat
- Chapped lips
- Moderate to severe dental caries (from binge-food selection)
- Pain
- Unaesthetic appearance of teeth

Many of the symptoms of anorexia and bulimia overlap, and it is not uncommon for an anorexic to also be bulimic. Table 15-1 compares symptoms of anorexia nervosa and bulimia nervosa. Figure 15-3 demonstrates the overlap in eating disorder symptoms.

🍎 **FOOD FOR THOUGHT 15-3**

University of Iowa researchers are proposing a new eating disorder called "purging disorder." It differs from bulimia in that the amount of food eaten is a very small amount. Bulimics gorge on food, consuming huge amounts, and then purge. Those with purging disorder limit their food intake and then vomit to maintain weight and body shape.

BINGE EATING

There is no mistaking a binge eater. They eat a great amount of food in a short period of time, usually by themselves. They eat until they are uncomfortably full, many times when they are not even hungry, and end up feeling disgusted,

TABLE 15-1   Symptoms of Anorexia and Bulimia

Symptom	Anorexia	Bulimia
Weight loss	×	
Weight fluctuation		×
Secretive eating		×
Binge eating		×
Fasting	×	×
Food obsession	×	
Use of laxatives	×	×
Use of diuretics	×	×
Use of diet pills	×	×
Purging		×
Heavy exercising	×	×
Wear inappropriate clothing	×	
Uncomfortable around food	×	
Frequent checking of weight	×	
Psychological depression	×	×
Low self-esteem	×	×
Withdrawn	×	
Guilt	×	×
Perfectionistic	×	
Physical Fatigue	×	×
Always cold	×	
Broken vessels		×
Swollen glands	×	×
Muscle weakness	×	×
Lanugo	×	

TABLE 15-1 *(continued)*

Symptom	Anorexia	Bulimia
Amenorrhea	×	×
Menstrual irregularities	×	×
Dizziness	×	×
Fainting	×	
Dehydration	×	×
Pallor	×	
Headaches	×	×
Dry skin and brittle hair	×	
Shortness of breath	×	×
Irregular heartbeats	×	×
Constipation	×	×
Low blood pressure	×	×
High blood pressure		×
Electrolyte imbalance	×	×
Chest pains		×
Gastric problems		×
Edema	×	×
Loss of bone mass	×	
Insomnia	×	
Anemia	×	×
Low potassium	×	
Cardiac arrest	×	×
Abrasions on index and middle finger		×
Death	×	×

depressed, and guilty for eating so much. The difference between the bulimic binging and the binge eater is that a binge eater does not purge, so all the calories end up making them obese. Obesity further complicates their life by adding risk for associated diseases. Binge eating is the most common of all eating disorders, affecting more individuals than all the other disorders combined.

Physical Symptoms of Binge Eating

- Obesity
- Diabetes
- High blood pressure
- High cholesterol
- Osteoarthritis
- Decreased mobility
- Shortness of breath
- Heart disease
- Liver and kidney problems
- Cardiac arrest
- Death

TREATMENT FOR EATING DISORDERS

Treatment for all eating disorders involves medical intervention, psychological help, and nutritional counseling. The sooner an eating disorder is diagnosed and treatment begins, more successful the intervention. Antidepressants are usually prescribed once weight has been stabilized.

Dental care is part of the recovery program. Oral effects of gastric acids and binging on cariogenic foods are usually the impetus for a visit to the dental office. Pain from erosion, dentinal sensitivity, and caries can get intense. Comprehensive dental treatment is usually postponed until behavior is changed so that tooth damage does not continue. Choice in restorative dental treatment depends on mental health status and the severity of damage to the teeth.

- Composites, overlays, crowns, and veneers can restore the teeth, depending on the severity of erosion.
- Fluoride and sodium bicarbonate rinses can prevent further sensitivity and enamel demineralization.
- Restoring the teeth to a more aesthetic appearance helps increase self-esteem.

See Food for Thought 15-4.

🍎 **FOOD FOR THOUGHT 15-4**

DENTAL TREATMENT

Aesthetic Restorations
- Crowns
- Composites
- Veneers

Home Care Instructions
- Wait 30 minutes after purging before brushing
- Rinse with sodium bicarbonate after purging
- Use a fluoride mouthwash before retiring for the night

Treatment for Sensitivity
- Use a toothpaste for sensitive teeth
- Use a commercially available desensitizing agent such as Protect, Seal and Protect, Duraflor, Pain-free, and so on

---

LESSER KNOWN EATING DISORDERS

- **Compulsive overeating**: uncontrollable eating and consequential weight gain. Food is used to comfort and de-stress. This is seen more frequently in males.
- **Anorexia athletica**: frantic exercising and fanatic about weight and diet. Time may be taken from school or work to exercise. People with this disease are rarely satisfied with physical achievements and move from one challenge to the next.
- **Body dysmorphic disorder**: excessively concerned about appearance and magnifies flaws. People with this body dysmorphic disorder may undergo multiple unneeded plastic surgeries.
- **Orthorexia nervosa**: excessive focus on eating pure or superior food. People with orthorexia nervosa usually obsess over what to eat and where to obtain it.
- **Pica**: craving and eating nonfood items such as dirt, laundry detergent, cigarette butts, clay, chalk, paint chips, cornstarch, baking soda, coffee grounds, glue, toothpaste, and soap. Pica may accompany a developmental disorder such as autism, mental retardation, or brain injury.

COUNSELING PATIENTS

[handwritten margin notes: dental erosion sensitivity asthetic problems]

The patient usually initiates a dental visit because of dental erosion, sensitivity, or aesthetic problems. The role of dental professional in treating patients with eating disorders is as follows:

- Case finding and referring to a medical professional
- Restoring dental and oral tissues
- Prevention

It is important to realize that a patient may relapse, so establishing regular recall visits to monitor dental care may prevent further damage. When counseling patients with an eating disorder, take care in how your instructions are worded. Their self-esteem is usually very fragile and if they perceive the visit as not going well, they will not continue treatment. Avoid placing blame or shame, using accusatory statements, and giving simple solutions to their dental problems. Express continued support, even if they have a relapse. Home care instructions should include the following:

[handwritten margin notes: baking soda magnesium hydroxide after vomiting]

- Rinse with water and baking soda or magnesium hydroxide after vomiting.
- Use home fluoride rinses before retiring for the night.
- Do not brush for 30 minutes after purging—allow saliva to remineralize enamel.
- Limit intake of acidic beverages.
- Avoid sticky, sweet foods between meals.
- Suck on sugar-free chewing gum or sugar-free hard candies (lemon balls) to stimulate saliva.
- Educate about the oral effects of purging:
  - Ditched amalgams
  - Enamel erosion
  - Sensitivity
  - Irregular incisal edges
  - Discolored teeth

Putting This Into Practice

1. Write out what you would say to a patient whom you suspect may be bulimic because of enamel erosion on the linguals of the maxillary anterior teeth and ditched amalgam fillings.

(continued)

2. If the client admits to bulimic purging, what wo
   prevention for further oral problems?
3. Research local eating disorder clinics and treatm
   notecard of addresses and phone numbers for
   accessed when needed.

WEB RESOURCES

Anorexia Nervosa and Related Eating Disorders http://www.anred.com/welcome.html

The National Eating Disorder Information Centre of Canada http://www.nedic.ca/

National Institute of Mental Health - Mental Disorders in America http://www.nimh.nih.gov/
   health/publications/the-numbers-count-mental-disorders-in-america.shtml

Academy for Eating Disorders http://www.aedweb.org/newwebsite/index.htm

Harvard Eating Disorders Center http://www.hedc.org/

National Eating Disorders Association
   http://www.nationaleatingdisorders.org/p.asp?WebPageID=337

The National Centre for Eating Disorders of the United Kingdom
   http://www.eating-disorders.org.uk/

Gurze Books—Eating Disorders Resources http://www.gurze.com/

Eating Disorder Referral and Information Center http://www.edreferral.com/

Overeaters Anonymous http://www.overeatersanonymous.org/

National Institute of Mental Health—Eating Disorders: Facts About Eating Disorders and
   the Search for Solutions http://www.nimh.nih.gov/publicat/eatingdisorders.cfm

National Women's Health Information Center—Body Image
   http://4women.gov/bodyimage/BodyImage.cfm?page=125

Body Positive—Boosting Body Image at Any Weight http://bodypositive.com

REFERENCES

1. Wöckel L, Jacob A, Holtmann M, et al. Reduced number of taste papillae in patients with eating disorders. *J Neural Transm* 2008;115(3):537–544.
2. Mond J, Myers TC, Crosby R, et al. Excessive exercise and eating disordered behavior in young women: further evidence from a primary care example. *Eur Eat Disord Rev* 2008.
3. Gavin J, Rodham K, Poyer H. The presentation of "pro-anorexia" in online group interactions. *Qual Health Res* 2008;18(3):325–333.

ayano M, Yoshiuchi K, Al-Adawi S, et al. Eating attitudes and body dissatisfaction in adolescents: Cross-cultural study. *Psychiatry Clin Neurosci* 2008;62(1):17–25.

SUGGESTED READING

Goldie MP. Striving for thin. *Dimens Dent Hyg* 2004:32–33.
Gurenlian JR. Eating disorders. *J Dent Hyg* 2002;76(3):219–234.

CHAPTER 16

NUTRITIONAL COUNSELING

OBJECTIVES

Upon completion of this chapter, the reader will be able to:

1 Understand the limits and boundaries of dental nutritional counseling
2 Identify a patient who would benefit from nutritional counseling
3 Discuss ways to incorporate nutritional counseling into a dental treatment plan
4 List assessment procedures that must be completed prior to nutritional counseling
5 Pick out clues in assessment data that would indicate the need for nutritional counseling as part of preventive treatment
6 Choose the best diet inventory for the patient's situation
7 Demonstrate nondirect counseling techniques to affect the best compliance
8 Offer well thought out suggestions to improve diet to keep the oral environment healthy

KEY TERMS

Direct Approach
Dysphagia
Nondirect Approach
Nutritional Referral

Open Body Language
24-Hour Recall
3-Day Diet Survey
7-Day Diet Survey

Computerized Diet Assessment

The American Dietetic Association recommends collaboration between dietetic and dental professionals to promote overall health as well as disease prevention and intervention. As research continues to establish solid links between oral and nutritional health, both professions must encourage their members to screen, educate, and refer to each other for total patient health.[1]

> It is fine for dental hygienists to give out general nutrition information, but state laws and licensure regulations draw the line when it comes to giving specific nutrition advice and counsel regarding a specific health condition. For that, oral health care professionals should refer patients to a registered dietitian. —*Gail Frank, DrPH, RD1*

Before getting started with nutritional counseling in the dental office, it is wise to understand the difference between what is expected of dental professionals and what is considered beyond the scope of practice. Dental nutritional counseling was developed to prevent or minimize dental disease and should be the goal in discussing food and diet with patients. Becoming involved in a patient's weight loss or recommending a diet for a specific medical condition is beyond the scope of practice and is better left to physicians or registered dietitians.

What do dental patients know? Most fail to recognize the relationship that nutritional status and eating habits have with their dental health. They do not really understand that what, when, and how they eat can affect their dental health. They do have a vague understanding that sugar causes cavities, but how diet relates to the health of the soft tissues and periodontium is not common knowledge. Teaching the interrelationship between diet and dental health can be as beneficial to the patient and as rewarding to the dental professional as teaching good home care.

There are many well-designed nutritional counseling forms on which to collect diet information; some have different layouts, but all will get you to the same end. If you do not have any forms or are unhappy with the ones you have, most dental and dental hygiene schools are very willing to share what they currently use. If your school or office is open to trying new ideas, visit the website of the school of choice and navigate. You can also visit the section at the end of this book to see if the nutritional counseling forms and instructions will work for you. Completing them yourself first allows you to get an idea of what you are asking your patients to do and how much time will need to be invested.

WHO CAN BENEFIT FROM DIETARY COUNSELING?

Almost everyone can benefit from learning something new and receiving information that can help improve his or her life. But certain groups are more at risk for nutritional deficiencies that cause or exacerbate dental disease. Knowing which groups to target can ensure that you are helping those with definite need. The following is a list of groups who can benefit from dental nutritional counseling:

- Elderly
  - The elderly are at high risk for dental caries because of salivary gland hypofunction and increased consumption of simple sugars. Buying food on a fixed income and preparing meals for one person are also complicating factors.
- Teenagers
  - Peer pressure for females to be thin or males to be muscular can create unusual eating habits. Convenience and fast foods are staples in the teen diet, and a balance in food choices is lacking in most cases.
- Bachelors
  - Bachelors are responsible only for themselves; meal planning and preparation is basically nonexistent.
- Adults who diet
  - Specialty diets may raise concerns. The grapefruit diet causes enamel erosion, and the Atkins diet eliminates carbohydrates, causing an imbalance in what is suggested by MyPyramid.
- Patients with change in dental health
  - New or recurrent caries can be a result of poor snack or meal choices. An increase in soda consumption and developing a new habit of sucking on hard candy can be devastating to enamel.
- Patients who take medications that cause a dry mouth
  - Lack of benefits from saliva can cause an increase in dental caries.

NUTRITIONAL COUNSELING AS PART OF PATIENT TREATMENT

In the Current Dental Terminology (CDT) 4 catalog, Nutritional Counseling (code D1310) is listed under Other Preventive Services. Unfortunately, there is no third party compensation for this procedure provided to dental practices. It falls into the same black hole as fluoride treatments or sealants for patients older than 14 years, which means to provide at the patient's expense. Because time equals money in the dental practice, the clinician may want to provide nutritional counseling during an appointment scheduled for another compensated procedure. Do not confuse an insurance company's lack of compensation for lack of importance. Preventive nutritional counseling is just as important during dental treatment as is reinforcing good home care.

The need for dental nutritional counseling is evaluated during the data collection phase of treatment. Procedures included in the data collection phase are as follows:

1. Medical/dental history
2. Vital signs
3. Intraoral/extra oral examination
4. Gingival examination
5. Periodontal Screening and Recording (PSR)/periodontal chart
6. Dental chart
7. Radiographs
8. Nutritional counseling

Clues to look for in the information obtained during data collection include the following:

- New or recurrent caries
- Tooth loss
- Skin lesions
- Atrophied lingual papillae
- Burning tongue
- Pale or gray mucosa
- Angular chelitis
- Greasy scaly skin around nose
- Inadequately functioning salivary glands
- Difficulty chewing or swallowing
- Ill-fitting dentures
- Sores under appliances
- Loss of lamina dura
- Polypharmacy (multiple medications)
- Erythemic marginal and attached gingiva
- Report of dietary change without physician supervision

If any of the above markers are discovered during data collection, the next step would be to explain the need for nutritional counseling to patients. Give patients a reason for wanting to participate. Explaining the relationship between what you found in their mouth to their diet is a great place to start. Initiating an open dialogue about food and snack selection can give the clinician insight into their eating habits. Once patients realize the connection between their diet and oral concern, their willingness for further investigation usually leads to informed consent. Patients have to be prepared and ready to make a change. Just as telling someone they need to quit smoking does not always cause the desired effect, neither will telling them to change their eating habits. They have to buy in to their need for change and be willing to work at it.

COLLECTING DIET INFORMATION

If it is determined that a patient can benefit from nutritional counseling and he or she is willing to participate, the next step is to gather information about his or her eating habits from a diet diary. There are several types of diet diaries to choose from:

- 24-hour recall
- 3-day food record
- 7-day food diary
- Computerized diet assessment

The **24-hour recall** works best if desiring a quick inquiry of a patient's eating habits. Simply ask the patient to list all the foods consumed in a 24-hour period, including amount and time of day eaten. Ask if it is a typical sample, and if not, ask what would make it typical. This can be accomplished while providing other treatment, while waiting for the dentist to give an examination, or after the dental charting. Although a form to record everything eaten in the course of a day is informative, quick target questions can be asked to determine the cariogenic potential of the diet if there are new carious lesions or erosion. If a patient reports sucking on breath mints or hard candy or sipping on four Diet Cokes in a day, you have probably discovered the source of new caries.

1. Do you drink either regular or diet soda or sweet tea?
2. Do you regularly drink fruit juice or sports drinks?
3. Do you suck on breath mints or hard candy?
4. Do you snack during the day, if so, how often?
5. Are the snacks usually sweet or sticky in nature?
6. Do you snack when you watch TV, play video games, and study?

7. Do you eat a lot of citrus fruits or drink citrus juices?
8. How many times a day and when do you brush and floss?

The **3- or 7-day diet diaries** is for a more in-depth study and should include at least 1 day of the weekend. This would require the patient to keep track of the food consumed on a daily basis. Forms should be explained and given to the patient to complete at home and return at the end of the week. After analyzing the content, appoint the patient for a one-on-one counseling session where deficiencies can be explained and suggestions for improvements made.

The **computerized diet assessment** is more general than dental related but is good for analyzing the nutrient content of food. There are several software programs that can be purchased or programs online that are helpful if a particular nutrient deficiency is suspected. A good place to start is at www.mypyramid.gov where a patient can customize their own food pyramid based on age, height, weight, and activity level.

UNDERSTANDING BARRIERS TO EATING WELL

Before counseling the patient, it is best to consider their lifestyle and determine if there are any barriers to eating well. Sometimes poor food choices are made for reasons other than lack of education. Certain lifestyle factors are beyond a patient's control and to not consider them may set both you and your patient up for failure. Be sure to inquire about daily eating patterns and ask open-ended questions about any concerns. When you have your answers, imagine yourself in their shoes and ask what you would do to improve eating habits. Provide suggestions that you are sure will fit into their lifestyle; otherwise you will be wasting a great opportunity to improve your patient's oral health.

- Many times job schedules dictate odd hours of eating.
- If patients live alone, does it make sense to prepare a three-course meal?
- Income plays a huge role in where a person shops and foods they choose. Organic produce and quality cuts of meat are expensive.
- Often single parents make choices as to whether they take a sick child to the doctor or dentist or buy food for the family for a week.
- Students in professional programs attend school from 9 AM to 5 PM and also try to work and study the remainder of the day.

- Convenience can be the single most important factor in choosing foods for busy families. Suggesting food choices that require time to prepare will fall on deaf ears. If they frequent fast-food restaurants, teach how to recognize and choose healthy items from the menu.

COUNSELING TECHNIQUES

When providing one-on-one counseling, there are basically two techniques or interactions:

- The **direct approach** is when you are the dictator and the patient plays a passive role. This is the most ineffective method because it is human nature to put up a defense when being told what to do. The directive to quit eating chocolate will fall on deaf ears every time. Figure 16-1 shows the patient in a passive role.
- With the **nondirect approach**, the patient is in control and the clinician's role is that of facilitator. This is also referred to the patient-centered technique. It demonstrates respect for what the patient already knows about his or her diet and nutrition, and allows for the patient's input and personal preferences. Change is more apt to happen via this method. Figure 16-2 shows the patient actively engaged in the discussion.

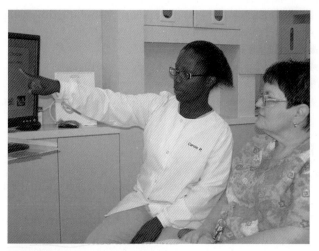

FIGURE 16-1   Direct approach.

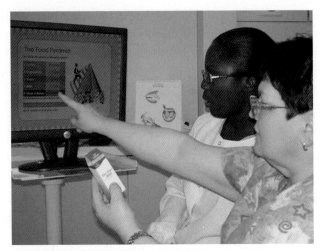

FIGURE 16-2   Nondirect approach.

Effective communication is a learned skill. The following are a few tips to make the counseling session more effective:

- Be nonjudgmental of current eating habits, likes, and dislikes.
- Let the patient know you are listening by engaging in good eye contact and nodding your head. Provide feedback as to what you understood them to say.
- Use **open body language**—no crossed arms, looking down, tapping pencils, swinging legs, or looking around.
- Offer encouragement.
- Sandwich criticism between two positive statements.
- Avoid finger pointing.
- Turn off or turn down the radio and block out external noises.

SETTING THE STAGE

Figures 16-3 and 16-4 show examples of food proportions that can be used to demonstrate your point.

It is best to counsel your patient in a place that does not invoke anxious feelings. Sitting at a table or counter is better than sitting in the treatment chair.

Seat patients at eye level and provide a surface where you can spread out their counseling forms and write, if necessary. Enhance the learning space with visual aids.

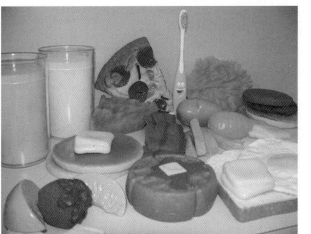

learn

75% vision
13% hearing
3% smell

FIGURE 16-3 **Food proportions.**

According to the Proctor and Gamble Dental Resource Net Adult Learning Online Program, we retain 75% of what we learn through the sense of vision, 13% through hearing, and 3% through taste and smell. Use the redireference card provided online as you provide information about healthy eating, snacks, and effect of foods on the oral cavity. Food for Thought 16-1 lists examples of visual aids.

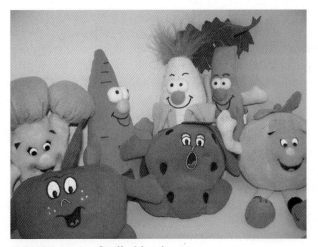

FIGURE 16-4 **Stuffed food toys.**

🍎 **FOOD FOR THOUGHT 16-1**

EXAMPLES OF VISUAL AIDS

- Laminated redireference card
  Food proportions
  Empty boxes and bottles of favorite foods
  Stuffed animal people
- Colorful Pyramid Guides
- Copy of the Guidelines for Americans (or other guidelines)
- Written changes patients have agreed to work on
- Written suggestions on how to make those changes

Need Guardian Children + Dependents

When counseling patients, there are two important considerations to keep in mind:

- If you counsel children, the parent has to be present.
- If you counsel a dependent person, the person responsible for his or her diet and preparing and serving his or her food must be present.

After the diet diary is returned and you have had time to examine it, ask yourself the following relative questions:

Analysis of the Diet Diary (see expanded step-by step suggestions on resource disc).

1. Did the patient meet the serving suggestions for the food groups in MyPyramid or other food guide (small or inactive people at the lower end and large or active at the upper end)?
2. Did the patient follow all points of the Dietary Guidelines chosen for them?
3. Did the patient minimize the minutes of acid attack each day?
4. Did the patient include one crunchy food per meal?
5. Did the patient include foods rich in nutrients that keep the periodontium healthy?

When Diet Changes Are Indicated

- Keep it simple.
- Make small changes.

- Offer no more than two suggestions at a time.
- Let the patient choose which two changes they want to work on.

When offering suggestions consider the following:

- Be consistent with current food habits, cultural influences, and regional preferences.
- Consider foods in season.
- Consider cost of food and patient's ability to pay for it.
- Make suggestions for choosing healthy meals at restaurants.
- Suggest changes to reduce cariogenic potential of diet.

WHEN TO REFER

Having the name of a respected doctor or nutritionist in your community will serve you well when it is determined a patient's nutritional counseling needs are beyond the scope of your practice and a **nutritional referral** would be in their best interest. If possible, introduce yourself to health care providers you will be referring to and explain your goals for future referrals. Open up a discussion of how nutrition plays a specific role in oral hygiene treatment and explain that a referral will be made when you suspect a disease process (other than caries and periodontal disease) is the result of poor nutrition.

When you believe a patient could benefit from a nutritional referral, discuss oral findings and their relationship with systemic disease first. Make sure the patient understands the relationship of their food choices and your concerns about their oral disease and how it may be contributing to other health concerns. This usually lays the foundation for understanding that your referral to a doctor or nutritionist will further improve their overall well being. The usual channel of referral is from doctor to registered nutritionist. The following list is just some of the reasons you might recommend a patient visit their doctor for nutritional advice:

- Improving heart health
- Suspected diabetes
- **Dysphagia**—difficulty swallowing
- Eating disorders
- HIV/AIDS
- Malnutrition
- Osteoporosis

COUNSELING PATIENTS

1. If a specific major nutrient deficiency or excess is discovered, such as protein, carbohydrates, or fats, include the suggestions for increasing the nutrient in the patient's diet listed at the end of those respective chapters.
2. If counseling to reduce cariogenicity of the diet, suggest limiting eating events to three times a day. Reduce snacking unless required for pregnancy or a medical condition.
3. If a patient snacks, recommend fresh fruits, vegetables, popcorn, yogurt, or cheese strips.
4. Cariogenic foods such as retentive starches and sugary foods/liquids should be consumed with meals.
5. When oral hygiene does not follow a meal or snack, suggest that the patient end the eating event with a dairy product, such as cheese or milk, or rinse thoroughly with water.
6. Discourage eating snacks before bed, unless followed by thorough brushing and flossing.
7. Include at least two to four servings of dairy products per day.
8. Drink water between meals and with snacks.
9. The protein and fat in meats cannot be metabolized by oral bacteria, so they have no impact on caries risk.
10. Cheese eaten at the end of a meal prevents pH from falling into the critical range.
11. Reinforce eliminating snack foods perceived as highly retentive.
    - Cookies
    - Crackers
    - Dry cereal
    - Potato chips
    - Caramels, jelly beans, and milk chocolate deliver high levels of sugar to bacteria immediately after the foods are consumed, but only for short periods of time.
12. Educate about the rate of oral clearance.
    - Process of dilution and elimination of food debris from the oral cavity: Normal salivary flow has a caries preventive effect by gradually diluting and removing carbohydrates from the mouth.
    - If meals or snacks are frequent, the calcium and phosphorus in saliva will not have a chance to remineralize the teeth between eating events, and a net demineralization results.

13. Suggest eating foods that stimulate saliva production. Eaten with a meal, they promote the buffering of acids produced by bacteria and clear food from the oral cavity.
    - Celery, carrots, raw broccoli and cauliflower, green pepper sticks
    - Sugar-free candy and gum
    - Apples and pears
14. Inform about foods that raise the salivary pH.
    - Cheese
    - Chicken
    - Pork
    - Beef
    - Fish
    - Dairy products
    - Chewing gum with xylitol
15. Educate on the physical forms of carbohydrates.
    - Liquid forms: fruit juice, sports drinks, coffee and tea if sugar is added, and soft drinks are in an acidic medium, which further demineralizes teeth.
    - Softening of enamel can occur in as little as 1 hour.
    - Diet sodas lower salivary pH and can demineralize tooth surfaces, independent of bacterial acid production.
16. More suggestions:
    - Replace diet and regular sodas with tea—unsweetened is best or add artificial sweetener (or fruit juice or water, if patients do not need caffeine).
    - Increase dairy products with yogurt, milk in cereal, or cheese added to a sandwich.
    - Switch to whole grains gradually by combining breads—one piece of white, one piece of whole-wheat—for a sandwich, with the white bread toward the tongue.
    - Gradually switch from whole milk to skim by drinking 2%, then 1%, then 0.5%, and finally skim milk.
    - Try mixing whole milk with 2% at first.
    - Vegetable and fruit juice is an excellent way to increase fruits and vegetables in the diet.
    - Select large pieces of fruit or take a larger portion of vegetables to increase serving size to equal two for each eating event.
    - Try mixing white and brown rice. Start with two tablespoon of brown rice per cup of white and gradually increase the ratio until brown rice predominates.

- Do not eliminate sweets if they are wanted; just eat them with meals.
- Try a healthy salad with dinner for crunchy food. The fiber will go a long way.
- Cereal is a quick way to increase grains and dairy products—and it is fortified.
- Frozen vegetables purchased in bags (do not forget to shake) are great for microwaving.
    — Most people have a tendency to eat the same foods for days, but vegetables in bags allow you to choose something different every day.
    — Just take out what you need and put the bag back in the freezer.

Putting This Into Practice

Complete a diet analysis on yourself using the forms provided in the forms section of this book. Follow the instructions for completion, analysis, and counseling. Take the following notes in a small notepad.

- Sections that seemed confusing
- Difficulties encountered in maintaining a daily log of foods consumed
- Questions that arose as you analyzed the food diary

WEB RESOURCES

Dietitians of Canada www.dieticians.ca

Government Nutrition Site www.nutrition.gov

REFERENCES

1. Decker R, Mobley C. Position of the American Dietetic Association: oral health and nutrition. *J Am Diet Assoc.* 2007;107(8):1418–1428.

SUGGESTED READING

Nappo-Dattoma, L. *Dental nutritional counseling techniques for the dental hygienist*. Accessed on, March 2008.

Altschuler B. Nutrition education the role of the dental hygienist. *Dental Hyg News* 1994;7(3).

Boyd LD, Dwyer JT. Guidelines for nutrition screening, assessment, and intervention in the dental office. *J Dent Hyg* 1998;72(4):31–43.

Dreizen S. Dietary and nutritional counseling in the prevention and control of oral disease. *Compendium* 1989;10(10):558–564.

Hackett AF, Rugg-Gunn AJ, Appleton DR. Use of dietary diary and interview to estimate the food intake of children. *Hum Nutr Appl Nutr* 1983;37(4):293–300.

Hornick B. Diet and nutrition implications for oral health. *J Dent Hyg* 2002;76(1):67–78.

Maclellan DL, Berenbaum S. Client-centered nutrition counseling: do we know what this means? *Can J Diet Pract Res* 2003;64(1):12–15.

Schneidhorst-Olson L. *The nutrition balancing act*. 1999.

CHAPTER 17

NUTRITIONAL COUNSELING FOR SPECIAL PATIENT GROUPS

OBJECTIVES

Upon completion of this chapter, the reader will be able to:

1 Identify special patient groups that may present for dental nutritional counseling
2 Discuss the influence of medical, dental, and lifestyle circumstances on nutritional counseling
3 Offer advice to patients on how to make eating more pleasant when they have xerostomia
4 List foods to avoid for patients with orthodontic appliances
5 Describe a healthy diet to keep the immune system healthy
6 Understand the diet limitations of someone who is homeless
7 Identify oral concerns of a patient living with HIV that may interfere with healthy eating
8 Counsel cancer patients on how to make their mouths more comfortable while eating

KEY TERMS

Cancer
Dental Surgeries
Developmental Disabilities
Diabetes
Human Immunodeficiency
  Virus (HIV)/Acquired

Immune Deficiency
  Syndrome (AIDS)
Homeless
Mucositis
Orthodontics
New Denture

Necrotizing Ulcerative Peri-
  odontal (NUP)
Substance Abuse
Temporomandibular Joint
  (TMJ)
Wounds

315

Life is rarely perfect. There will be times when you find yourself in a situation where your patient requires nutritional counseling but their life circumstances are complicated or different than the accepted norm. Just as we do not give the same exact oral hygiene instructions to every patient we treat, we do not give the same nutritional counseling advice to each patient in need. Presentations are tailored to specific oral concerns, assessment findings, physical and mental ability, patient's likes and dislikes, and lifestyle/living arrangements. Dental specialty practices may offer specific diet recommendations before and after treatment and some medical concerns require diet modifications. There are also times when a patient needs our expert guidance while trying to improve their living situation, whether their current address is a local shelter or they are recovering from a life-threatening addiction. Knowing the specific nutritional concerns as well as which foods to suggest for the situation, help us give wise counsel for healing and repair of oral tissues, or prevention of oral disease.

As a dental healthcare professional, you owe it to each patient to understand them as a "whole" person. If they have a chronic disease or diagnosed disability, research the condition with a depth and breadth you would appreciate if you were standing in their shoes. Visit reliable websites, research professional publications, or add to your personal research library with book purchases on related disorders. I would encourage you to keep an indexed binder filled with current articles on the various diseases/disorders and their oral concerns in your operatory or office library so you will have the data available on short notice.

WOUND HEALING CONCEPTS

In the practice of dentistry, we see oral wounds on a daily basis. The **wounds** have many origins, which can be the result of a disease process, surgery, neglect, or treatment. Periodontal disease is a wound, which occurs as a result of chronic bacterial infection. Traumatic injuries can tear, cut, avulse teeth, and fracture bone. Elective oral or periodontal surgery can leave open tooth sockets, raw denuded tissue, incisions, and other situations that require tissue and bone to heal. Heavy scaling and root smoothing can inadvertently peel the inside lining of periodontal pockets, requiring the body to generate new epithelial tissue. Whatever the reason for oral wounds, a need for tissue to heal and repair will require a change in diet. Knowledge of those needs is required by the healthcare provider before giving sound nutritional advice.

One of the best things a patient can have going for them is a strong immune system to stave off infection and repair tissue in a timely manner. Stress, infections, and tissue injuries require an increase in all nutrients. Recommending specific nutrients that keep immune systems functioning properly will assure proper healing.

- When the body is wounded, there is a 25% increase in total caloric requirement for metabolic function that assists with healing and repairing activities.
- If body temperature is elevated, there is a 12% increase in nutrient requirement for every degree of elevation.
- Adequate dietary protein is needed for making new tissue and if there is a deficiency, the body will draw from its own structures (muscle).
- Recommendations for adequate caloric intake should be made so the body has the energy requirement necessary for metabolic processes.
- Vitamin C and Zinc assist with wound healing
- B Complex vitamins keep the immune system healthy

Oral/Maxillofacial and Periodontal Surgery Patient

Dental surgeries include tooth extraction, site biopsy, orthognathic surgery, repair of facial trauma, bone grafting, crown lengthening, dental implants, gingivoplasty, gingival tissue graft, and pocket reduction. If not for pain medication, all postoperative surgery patients would feel significant pain in the area of operation. A wound has been created and will take time to heal. There is an increased need for total caloric intake, and many specialty practices will recommend some type of liquid supplementation such as Ensure or Sustical. Solid foods can also be eaten as long as the patient feels comfortable, but if hard to tolerate, soft foods should be eaten for 3 to 4 days until *significant* healing has occurred. The following is a list of foods to *avoid* for the first 3 to 5 days after surgery:

- Spicy foods
- Salty foods
- Crunchy or hard foods
- Excessively hot foods and beverages
- Alcoholic beverages

If oral surgery involved tooth extraction, the following additional diet recommendations should be suggested:

- Avoid smoking and sucking through a straw because this can dislodge the blood clot and a painful dry socket occurs
- Drink plenty of fluids

- Eat only soft foods during the first 12 to 24 hours
- Chew on the opposite side of the wound

Necrotizing Ulcerative Periodontal Disease

Necrotizing ulcerative periodontal (**NUP**) disease is a destructive infection that causes necrosis of gingival tissues accompanied by bone loss. Tissues are fiery red, bleed spontaneously, and are extremely painful. Patients will present with elevated temperatures and lymphadenopathy and report a sense of lethargy. Dental treatment consists of aggressive debridement, patient education, and nutritional counseling. The following are diet suggestions that can help the patient through the first few critical days of healing:

- Increase caloric intake as required because of fever and need for tissue repair
- Have a liquid or soft diet for the first few days
- Avoid all spicy or irritating foods
- Choose bland floods that feel soothing, such as gelatin, ice cream, apple-sauce, and pudding
- Eat frequent small meals
- Drink plenty of fluids
- Take vitamin/mineral supplements as recommended by the dentist

CHEWING CONSIDERATIONS

Successfully chewing food is completely taken for granted by those with a healthy natural dentition because they have no idea what it is like to try to chew with few or no teeth or to chew when each movement causes pain. Tooth loss, mobility, jaw pain, and oral appliances will limit the ability to tear and grind and can have an affect on whether one chooses nutritious foods.

New Dentures

In the mid 1950s, the majority of Americans older than 65 years were edentulous. Improvements in high-speed handpieces and use of local anesthetics changed the trend by making dental restorations pain-free and more attractive. Then with the advent of dental insurance in the 1970s, it was financially possible for millions more to accept tooth restoration as the treatment of choice instead of extraction.[1] Water fluoridation further reduced tooth loss through caries prevention. Despite our best efforts through education and improvements in dental technology, we still see patients, to this day, with missing or mobile teeth because of oral neglect. And with the rising cost of dental services, some patients will insist on a less expensive extraction than a more expensive root canal and crown or implant. If a healthy diet is directly related to ability to chew, then the more teeth present, the better ability to chew, and better nutrition.

Chewing (grinding food) with natural teeth can deliver a force of approximately 200 lb per square inch. Dentures are only 25% as effective. Put yourself in this scenario: You want to eat raw carrots, corn on the cob, and steak. Your palate is completely covered with a piece of hard plastic. You are trying to bite into the steak with your front teeth and grind with your back molars, but biting and grinding does not work like it used to be. Tearing food with the front teeth feels like the denture can be pulled right out of the mouth along with the food. And grinding feels more like smashing the food and it just does not pulverize as well as natural teeth, therefore, you have to swallow big chunks of food, which are hard to digest. You wonder why you did not take better care of your teeth. As the saying goes, you don't appreciate what you have until it is gone.

The **new denture** patient has to learn to talk and chew in a new way and the dental healthcare professional can help them accept the limitation of new dentures as they adjust to the "rules for eating." The following is a list of diet suggestions that may be helpful during this time of change:

- Know that food will not taste the same—flavors are masked by the denture
- Cut regular food into small pieces
- Chew food on both sides with the back teeth to prevent tipping of the denture
- Take small bites and chew slowly
- Start with soft foods such as eggs, fish, cooked vegetables, and pudding
- Avoid sticky or very hard foods in the beginning
- Be careful with hot food and drink as the covered palate will protect against high temperatures and the heat will not be felt until the food or drink hits the esophagus on its way down

Temporomandibular Joint Disorder

Experiencing pain in the temporomandibular joint (**TMJ**), one of the most frequently used and most complex joints in the body, can decrease quality of life. According to the American Dental Association, 15% of American adults experience TMJ disorder at one point in their lives with greater incidence reported in women then men. Causes of this disorder can be from injury or trauma, tension and stress, poor tooth alignment, arthritis, and tumors. Problems with this joint can involve the muscles, ligaments, bone, or disc. Pain from this joint can be referred to the ear, face, and neck causing migraine-like headaches, earaches, and pain behind the eyes. Patients report annoying popping and clicking when opening, yawning, or chewing, and sometimes the jaw will get stuck in a certain position.

Degeneration of the joint will cause pain upon chewing. Learning to manage pain while eating is important as the patient collaborates with the dental professional for permanent relief. The following are suggestions that can be made that are helpful in alleviating pain while chewing:

- Avoid foods that require you to open wide. Chewing ability is limited to how wide the mouth can open and close. Some patients will try to compress foods that are stacked higher than they can open, like a Big Mac or deli sandwich.
- If the smallest movements during chewing are painful, liquid supplements like Ensure and Sustical offer all needed nutrients and calories.
- A soft diet is best with eating events divided into several small meals a day so the amount of time needed to chew in one sitting is limited.

Orthodontic Appliances

The main concern about diet and **orthodontics** is that some foods will displace the brackets, loosen cement under bands, and bend the ligature wire. Plaque accumulates around appliances and is awkward to remove. If the patient has frequent eating episodes of carbohydrates, there is a greater opportunity for acid production and enamel demineralization. The patient should be instructed to avoid eating hard or sticky foods and those with high carbohydrate content. Most foods can be eaten, but they should be cut into bite-sized pieces. Teeth are usually sore after adjustments so soft foods are tolerated best. Prepare ahead for adjustment days by planning snacks and meals of soft consistency. Examples of foods to avoid are as follows:

- Popcorn (especially kernels), nuts, and peanut brittle
- Ice
- Corn on the cob
- Sticky candy such a gummy bears, caramels, taffy, and jelly beans
- Any kind of soda
- Corn chips and crispy tacos
- Chewing gum
- Hard bagels, bread, rolls, or pizza crust
- Lemons

- Hard pretzels
- Whole pieces of fruit (cut into small pieces)

MEDICAL DISORDERS

Providing nutritional counseling to dental patients for prevention of dental caries or improving periodontal health when they have a diagnosed medical condition is slightly more involved than counseling those with good general health. A good understanding of the medical disorder and any related digestive or nutritional irregularities will allow you to make suggestions that would be approved by the physician. This is where having current information and the latest research about the disorder comes in handy.

We are taught in school that each time a patient presents for treatment, their medical history is updated, and few are the numbers of those completing a form without any positive responses. Regardless of what is revealed on the medical history, we are responsible for providing wise nutritional counseling for prevention of dental caries and maintenance of good periodontal health. Having consideration for their medical diagnoses, while counseling on dental health, will greatly improve compliance with nutritional suggestions.

Diabetes

Millions of people have been diagnosed with **diabetes**, and there may be millions more who have symptoms but are not yet diagnosed. Following are the three main types of diabetes:

- Type 1: autoimmune destruction of the cells that produce insulin in the pancreas
- Type 2: impaired insulin function
- Gestational: glucose intolerance during pregnancy (usually temporary situation)

It is estimated that 20% of all adults older than 65 years are diabetic. Ninety-five percent of diabetics have type 2 diabetes.[2,3] With figures like these, it is more than likely that dental professionals will treat many diabetic patients in their practice. The following are some risks for an increased chance of developing diabetes:

- Prolonged hyperglycemia
- Advancing age
- Obesity

- Long-term lack of physical exercise
- Hypertension
- Genetic predispositio
  - African American
  - Hispanic
  - Native American

For those who are healthy, insulin helps bodies maintain blood sugar levels. Our pancreas secretes insulin when there is an excess of glucose in our blood, such as after a carbohydrate rich meal, and removes the surplus of glucose, storing it in the muscle and liver as glycogen, where it can be accessed for future energy use. This process of insulin production and glucose removal is ineffective in diabetic patients. Dental management of diabetic patients should include the following:

- Obtaining a thorough and accurate medical history
- Inquiring about self-management of the disease:
  - Oral medications, including dosage and times
  - Eating patterns
  - Insulin injections
  - Frequency of blood glucose readings
- Educating about oral manifestations
  - Oral burning if uncontrolled
  - Increased incidence of periodontal disease
    — Diabetic patients have a severalfold greater incidence of periodontal disease
  - Xerostomia because of decreased function of parotid gland
    — Increased dental caries at gingival third
    — Angular chelitis and candida infection because of low salivary flow

When providing nutritional counseling in the dental setting for the diabetic patient, be reminded that it is beyond the scope of the dental practice to give counseling advice for a specific medical condition. Advising for a diet that can reduce dental caries and periodontal disease are within the bounds of a dental healthcare worker and may be necessary if these conditions exist. The following should be included when counseling a diabetic patient:

- Sip on water or chew sugarless gum to help alleviate dry mouth and stimulate saliva flow
- Follow a balanced diet as prescribed by the physician/dietitian to ensure adequate nutrient intake

- Add a multivitamin to daily regimen, if not already doing so
- Include cariostatic foods where allowed in the daily diet
- Practice thorough daily plaque removal with sulcular brushing and some type of interproximal aid

Cancer

Cancer is a type of disease where body tissue cells act abnormally; they divide and grow in an uncontrolled way, which then invade and destroy tissue. As of 2007, estimated new cases for all types of cancer are 1,444,000. Good nutrition is important before and after treatment because the disease and treatments can alter desire for and ability to tolerate certain foods, and the body's ability to absorb nutrients. A debilitated body is more prone to infection and will not heal and repair as well. Cancer patients can be proactive by eating the right type of food so they can feel their best before, during, and after treatment. There is a need for increase in total caloric consumption as well as good lean protein, but some of the side effects of cancer treatment make it hard to eat. It is very common to experience loss of appetite, difficulty swallowing, mouth ulcers, nausea, constipation, and diarrhea. Another common complaint that stems from altered taste and smell is a metallic taste in the mouth. Rinsing the mouth with baking soda and water before eating or using plastic eating utensils, or eating fresh fruits and vegetables versus those in a can will offer some relief. Two side-effect complaints that may bring a patient with cancer to the dental office are xerostomia and mouth ulcers.

Xerostomia can be a problem if treatment involves medications that dry out the mouth or if radiation to the head and neck diminishes salivary output. Suggestions for these patients for prevention of dental caries would be:

- Eat moist foods with extra sauce, gravy, and butter
- Suck on sugar-free hard candy and chew gum with xylitol
- Eat frozen fruit like berries, melon, and grapes or all fruit popsicles
- Sip on water throughout the day and rinse your mouth often
- Use a straw for most beverages to bypass vulnerable teeth
- Choose fruit nectar instead of juice as it is less acidic

Chemotherapy and radiation therapy to the head and neck can cause painful, bleeding mouth ulcers that can last as long as treatment continues. The following are helpful suggestions for these patients:

- Eat soft foods like canned fruit, pudding, applesauce, cottage cheese, mashed potatoes, scrambled eggs, pasta, oatmeal or cream of wheat cereal, and jello

- Puree meats and vegetables
- Avoid spicy and salty foods
- Avoid any food that has vinegar such as pickles and salad dressing
- Avoid foods that have citric acid such as lemons, oranges, grapefruits, and limes
- Cut food into small bite-sized pieces
- Avoid dry foods such as crackers, toast, and granola
- Numb the mouth with ice chips

Human Immunodeficiency Virus/Acquired Immune Deficiency Syndrome

According to the Center for Disease Control's Surveillance Report there are more than 33 million people suffering from **HIV/AIDS** in the world, 1.2 million in the United States. HIV is the virus that causes the AIDS disease by destroying the immune system, making it impossible for an infected individual to fight off disease and infections. The U.S. Department of Veteran's Affairs has a photo library of oral manifestations of HIV/AIDS: http://www.hiv.va.gov/vahiv?page=im-1-04 which can help the dental healthcare worker identify oral complications of the disease in patients. There are many oral manifestations of the disease that are of concern to the dental healthcare worker including necrotizing periodontitis, candida, kaposi sarcoma, and aphthous ulcers, all of which can make chewing and swallowing painful. Side effects of a cocktail of medication are anorexia, nausea, and xerostomia. Many AIDS patients will eat a diet high in simple carbohydrates for taste and palatability when their desire for food is minimal. Comfort foods like milkshakes, pudding, and ice cream help keep energy levels high when there is no appetite for other foods. The danger in that practice is it puts them at a higher risk for dental caries.

Many immunocompromised patients seek dental treatment to help alleviate the oral symptoms of bleeding, **mucositis** (painful inflammation and ulceration of mucosa), periodontal infection, or restoration of carious teeth. Treatment for prevention of caries and periodontal disease should be aggressive. Frequent oral hygiene therapy visits and fluoride treatments are recommended.

General nutritional counseling suggestions for dental patients with HIV/AIDS should include staying well hydrated, increasing total caloric intake fortified with plenty of good lean sources of protein. Liquid dietary supplements are excellent to fortify insufficient diets. Patients should be educated about the carious process and a caries reduction diet should be recommended.

For specific help with mucositis, patients can be counseled to do the following:

- Suck on ice to numb tissues
- Eat a bland diet (no spice)

- Puree solid foods
- Avoid alcohol

For xerostomia, try the oral lubricators before recommending the one you feel works best. Counsel to do the following:

- Sip on water
- Eat foods with extra sauce, gravy, and butter
- Suck on sugar-free hard candy
- Chew sugar-free gum

DEVELOPMENTAL DISORDERS

The Center for Disease Control defines **developmental disabilities** as a group of severe chronic conditions caused by mental and/or physical impairments that impedes life activities such as language, mobility, learning, self-help, and independent living. Not all are discovered at time of birth as they can develop up to 22 years of age. Autism, cerebral palsy, vision and hearing impairment, Down syndrome, and Fragile X are examples of developmental disorders. There is no cure, but educational programs can teach individuals and their caregivers how to maximize the faculties they were given. Oral concerns of children with developmental disabilities are not any different than for children without disabilities.[4,5] Both children and adults with development disabilities are at no higher risk for dental caries than the general population, but for various reasons unique to their group, they can be considered high risk: inadequate oral hygiene because of poor eye-hand motor control, infrequent dental visits, trouble accessing care due to special transportation needs, higher percentage of malocclusion, and financial considerations.

Parents who care for children with developmental disabilities may have them follow a specific diet which may or may not have a scientific foundation. Some proponents favor special diets for autistic children—avoid gluten and casein (wheat and dairy) thinking it causes foggy thinking and food cravings. Also gastrointestinal complaints are not uncommon. Suggest foods easy to digest, rich in good bacteria, naturally fermented bacteria (yogurt), and pureed vegetables. It is best not to interfere with what a parent feels is best for their child and is a conversation better left to the nutritionist or physician. However, educating about the process of dental caries and explaining the role nutrients have in maintaining healthy periodontium can only improve the diet they currently follow.

Many adults with developmental disabilities live in a group home with others who may have a different disability. Social services have organized educational programs that teach disabled individuals about good nutrition and will even provide lessons on how to prepare healthy meals. Patients with developmental disabilities often choose easy foods—finger food, ready made, and store bought food, which do not take a lot of time, steps, or ingredients to prepare. Finding out what their favorite foods are or what they eat most often is the first step in determining a diet that sustains oral health. If their favorite food is cariogenic, offer a healthier substitution. For example, if they eat donuts everyday, encourage them to eat cold cereal with milk. If they drink soda, suggest tea sweetened with sugar substitute. Talk about colors on a plate—the more colors the healthier; for example, green and orange vegetables, piece of meat, and sliced tomatoes instead of one large bowl of macaroni and cheese. Keep the sessions simple and aim for small changes.

LIFESTYLE CONCERNS

Stop and think about your life right at this moment. Do you know where you will sleep tonight? Are you sure there will be food for your next meal? Do you go about the day's activity without the need for alcohol or drugs? If you have answered "yes" to all three of these questions, consider yourself among the lucky. But chances are there was a time in your life that you would have answered "no" to one or more of the questions. Whether we like it or not, our patients, like us, have very complex lives that are in a constant state of flux. Daily stressors from demands put upon us and limited time can make us callous in a moment when we need to be our softest. Understanding that patients are not always where they want to be in their lives when they present for treatment can make us call upon our more empathetic nature. Nutritional advice needs to be practical for all aspects of life. It is not a good idea to suggest patients eat more fresh fruit and vegetables when they get their food from a dumpster. It makes no sense to tell a mother to feed her young child milk when she has no means to keep it cold from one meal to the next. And a drug addict is more concerned about when they can make their next score, not where they can find fresh carrots to snack on.

Homeless Patients

The National Coalition for the Homeless (http://www.nationalhomeless.org/publications/facts/How_Many.pdf) estimates 3.5 million Americans, including 1.35 million children (half of them younger than 6 years), are **homeless** at one point in their lives. Extended unemployment, domestic abuse, increased cost of housing and few choices for affordable housing, as well as natural disasters all factor in to individuals and families forced to live in their cars, on the street, or shelters. Exact statistics for homelessness are difficult to obtain because the numbers fluctuate on any given night and there are certain homeless groups that remain hidden. Runaway teenagers who fear being sent home or families who double up with relatives and friends are not present at shelters and soup kitchens when heads are being counted. There are two groups of homeless—the long-term homeless, such as those who suffer from mental illness, drug, or gambling addiction, and temporary homeless who find themselves without shelter and are suddenly pushed into a new culture. The long-term homeless are pretty savvy at finding places to sleep and eat on the street but the short-term or newly homeless need time to figure out resources until their luck changes.

Food security is a primary issue for the homeless; inability to store or cook food eliminates that reliable feeling of knowing where the next meal is coming from. Strategies used to secure food are soup kitchens, food stamps, stealing food, eating food in grocery stores, pawning personal items, using savvy shopping habits, scavenging in dumpsters, and sacrificing food for children.[6] Studies show many homeless have the knowledge and desire to eat healthy but have a problem accessing affordable healthier food.[7]

See Food for Thought 17-1 and 17-2.

🍎 FOOD FOR THOUGHT 17-1

According to the U.S. Census Bureau, 5 million adults and 2.7 million children lived in hungry households. A poor diet in early childhood has implications for long-term health and cognitive development.

🍎 FOOD FOR THOUGHT 17-2

"Most shelters rely on private donations, a local food bank, and surplus commodity distributions. Because the nutritional quality and quantity of these resources vary greatly over time, meals may be nutritionally limited, even though the quantity of the food served may be acceptable to the recipient" (Wolgemuth et al., 1992, 834).

Homeless individuals have considerable oral health needs with two third of a research sample reporting some type of facial pain over the last year.[8] One of the last things a homeless person is concerned about is receiving preventive dental care, but they will seek palliative treatment for pain. Some community shelters have financial resources to assist residents with medical and oral healthcare needs. One of the main objectives of social services is to assist individuals to become employed, and being free from pain and having a nice smile will go a long way at an interview.

Time may not allow for a formal nutritional counseling process, as it is difficult to schedule subsequent appointments and cost is a factor. But a 24-hour diet recall or open-ended discussion about foods eaten the previous 3 days can be a great starting point for a discussion on good nutrition. Nutritional counseling advice for the homeless should include suggestions for overall general health, prevention of dental caries, benefits of foods that bring saliva into the mouth, and foods with nutrients that assist with healing and keeping the immune system healthy.

Substance Abuse

Mind altering drugs, alcohol, and tobacco are the three most abused substances. Abuse is simply overindulgence in a substance that if used long enough will cause harm to the mind and body. **Substance abuse** may or may not lead to addiction. Addiction, also referred to as "dependence," occurs when a physiological need for the substance develops; there is a gradual tolerance requiring increased amounts to get desired effect and withdrawal symptoms when use is stopped. When addicted, an individual will experience mental and physical cravings that occur from substance residues that stay in the body long after the last episode of use. Addiction is a disease for which there is no absolute cure; addicted individuals simply go into remission and learn to manage the cravings and urges to start using again.

Oral health needs of individuals with an addiction stem from poor oral hygiene and neglect, bruxism, and poor diets that consist mainly of simple carbohydrates. During recovery, patients may use food as a substitute for their craving for drugs or alcohol. They give in to binge eating, gain weight, and then struggle with establishing normal eating patterns. Nutritional counseling for those in recovery should include suggestions for overall good health:

- Take a daily multivitamin/mineral supplement
- Help set routine schedules for meals
- Establish parameters for between meal snacking
- Counsel about the caries process and help eliminate barriers to keeping the potential acid production less than 60 minutes a day
- Suggest foods that will stimulate saliva production
- Chew gum with xylitol

According to the 2003 National Survey on Drug Use and Health, more than 12 million Americans have tried methamphetamine, a central nervous system (CNS) stimulant that has similar physical and psychological effects to cocaine. Effects of the drug elicit a sense of euphoria, exceptional energy, increased attention, decreased fatigue, and a sense of invulnerability. Anorexia is one of the side effects of the methamphetamine abuse, and because of nonstop movement, users will look emaciated and undernourished. "Meth-mouth" is an accepted term to describe a cluster of oral finding on someone who abuses the drug:

- Fast developing rampant caries (within a year)
- Stained and crumbling teeth
- Tooth fracture and muscle trismus from bruxing
- Tooth loss
- Enamel erosion
- Xerostomia

One study found that methamphetamine users were more likely to snack without eating defined meals, consume regular soda, never brush their teeth, and smoke than were nonusers.[9] The problem with rampant caries in methamphetamine users results mainly from xerostomia caused by the acidic nature of the drug, increase in soda consumption because of carbohydrate craving, and lack of oral hygiene. Visit http://www.ada.org/public/topics/methmouth.asp to learn what the American Dental Association has to say about meth-mouth.

It is usually seeking relief from oral pain that brings methamphetamine abusers to the dental office. When they do present, they may not be open to recommendations for cessation of drug abuse, but it is an opportune time to talk with them about the process of dental caries and make suggestions for small changes in their diet. As long as the patient continues to abuse methamphetamines, it is difficult for future appointments so complete nutritional counseling may not be possible. A 24-hour diet recall can identify the most destructive diet habits and can open a conversation on how to mitigate the damages. The following are some diet changes that may be easy to implement and accepted by the patient:

- Drink tea with artificial sweeteners instead of soda
- Drink one can of flavored diet supplement per day (Ensure or Sustical) instead of soda
- Sip on water and rinse the mouth often

When the patient is in recovery, suggestions for general nutritional health should be made.

Putting This Into Practice

1. Choose two of the special patient groups and make information sheets for your dental practice to give the client as take home instructions. Include the following:
   a. Description of the service just provided at the office
   b. What to expect in the next 24 hours
   c. Suggestions of foods to avoid
   d. Suggestions of foods to include in the diet
   e. Any special oral care instructions
2. Make a list of referral agencies to use as a resource for patients.
   a. Include organizations that serve free meals
   b. Alcoholics Anonymous and Alanon
   c. Homeless shelters
   d. Shelters for battered women
   e. Shelters that accept families
   f. Contacts at public schools to sign-up children for free breakfast and lunch

WEB RESOURCES

Estimated new cancer cases and deaths by sex for all sites
http://www.cancer.org/downloads/stt/CFF2007EstCsDths07.pdf

Center for Disease Control and Prevention
http://www.cdc.gov/hiv/resources/factsheets/index.htm#Surveillance

US Dept of Health and Human Services Statistics on Substance Abuse
http://www.drugabusestatistics.samhsa.gov/newpubs.htm

Alcoholics Anonymous http://www.alcoholics-anonymous.org/?Media=PlayFlash

ARC of the United States http://www.thearc.org/NetCommunity/Page.aspx?&pid=217&srcid=268&txtSearch=how+many+disabled+in+america

REFERENCES

1. Ecklund SA. Changing treatment patterns. *J Am Dent Assoc* 1999;130(12):1707–1711.
2. Lalla RV, D'Ambrosio JA. Dental management considerations for the patient with diabetes mellitus. *J Am Dent Assoc* 2001;132(10):1425–1432.

3. American Diabetes Association. Position statement on evidence based nutrition principles and recommendations for the treatment and prevention of diabetes and related complications. *Diabetes Care* 2002;25(1):202–212.

4. Kopycka-Kedzierawaski DT, Auinger P. Dental needs and status of autistic children: results from the National Survey of Children's Health. *Pediatr Dent* 2008;30(1):54–58.

5. DeMattei R, Cuvo A, Maurizio S. Oral assessment of children with an autism spectrum disorder. *J Dent Hyg* 2007;81(3):65.

6. Richards R, Smith C. The impact of homeless shelters on food access and choice among homeless families in Minnesota. *J Nutr Educ Behav* 2006;38(2):96–105.

7. Wicks R, Trevena LJ, Quine S. Experiences of food insecurity among urban soup kitchen consumers: insights for improving nutrition and well-being. *J Am Diet Assoc* 2006;106(6): 921–924.

8. Conte M, Broder HL, Jenkins G, et al. UMDNJ-New Jersey Dental School, Department of Community Health, Oral health, related behaviors and oral health impacts among homeless adults. *J Public Health Dent* 2006;66(4):276–278.

9. Morio KA, Marshall TA, Qian F, et al. Comparing diet, oral hygiene and caries status of adult methamphetamine users and nonusers: a pilot study. *J Am Dent Assoc* 2008;139(2): 171–176.

SUGGESTED READING

Grosso G, Prajer R. Substance use and its impact on Dental Hygiene treatment. *J Public Health* 2007:22–24.

Nanne S. Salivary substitutes and oral lubricants—providing patient with relief from xerostomia. *J Public Health* 2007:17–19.

Seidel-Bittke D. Caring for the developmentally disabled. *RDH* 2005;32:34,36.

Making a PowerPoint Presentation Specific for Your Patient's Needs

1. Click on the following link and complete the boxes using your patient information http://www.mypyramid.gov/mypyramid/index.aspx
2. Save the address in the url and copy it to a powerpoint slide. For example: http://www.mypyramid.gov/mypyramid/results.html?name=undefined&age=55&gender= female&weight=130&heightfeet=5&heightinch=3&activity=sed&weightN= 126&heightfeetN=5&heightinchN=3&validweight=1&validheight=1&
3. Click on "Inside the Pyramid" on the menu to the left and save the address in the url and copy it to a powerpoint slide. http://www.mypyramid.gov/pyramid/index.html
4. Navigate by clicking on each colored section of the pyramid to educate your patient about the value of each food group
5. Click on the first food item in blue font OR use the links on the following page to educate as to what constitutes a serving size in each of the food groups.
6. Click on the physical activity link in the related topics menu to see a chart of physical activity.
7. Include slides on dental caries and/or periodontal disease. If your school does not have a common library of pictures, there are many on public domain websites that you can borrow.

The following web pages off the www.mypyramid.gov website have pictures and charts that can be incorporated into PowerPoint presentation individualized for your patient's needs. Right click on the picture and save it to a folder on your desktop. Then insert in your PowerPoint presentation.

What counts as an ounce of grain?
    http://www.mypyramid.gov/pyramid/grains_counts_table.html
How does a serving size of vegetables look like
    http://www.mypyramid.gov/pyramid/food_library/vegetables/carrots.html
How does a serving size of fruit looks like
    http://www.mypyramid.gov/pyramid/food_library/fruit/apples.html
How does a serving size of dairy product looks like
    http://www.mypyramid.gov/pyramid/food_library/milk/skim.html
How does a serving size of meat looks like
    http://www.mypyramid.gov/pyramid/food_library/meat/lean_beef.html
Information's on oils
    http://www.mypyramid.gov/pyramid/oils.html
Chart on physical activity
    http://www.mypyramid.gov/pyramid/calories_used_table.html

GLOSSARY

A

acid production—a period during the caries process when bacteria secrete acid

alveolar bone—bone of the human skull that contains the tooth sockets

amino acid—a molecule containing both an amine and carboxyl group

ana—modern abbreviation for anorexia nervosa eating disorder

anion—negatively charged ion

antidiuretic hormone (ADH)—hormone released by the pituitary gland that has an antidiuretic action that prevents the production of dilute urine

antioxidant—substance that reduces damage to cells caused by free radicals attaching oxygen to molecules

B

B-complex—group of several B vitamins

binge—unrestrained excessive indulgence

bioavailability—rate at which a substance is absorbed into a living system or is made available at the site of physiological activity

biologic value—measure of proportion of absorbed protein from food that gets incorporated into the body

C

calcium—major mineral predominant in dairy products used by the body for formation of strong teeth and bones

caries equation—plaque bacteria + fermentable carbohydrate = acid production, which demineralizes teeth

caries risk—high or low potential for developing dental caries

cariogenic—ability to contribute to formation of dental caries

cariostatic—does not contribute to the initiation or development of dental caries

cations—positively charged ion

CHO—abbreviation for carbohydrate

chylomicron—a lipoprotein rich in triglyceride and common in the blood during fat digestion and assimilation

collagen—fibrous proteins in connective tissue

complementary protein—a protein that is incomplete by itself, but together with another protein will provide all the amino acids for a complete protein

complete protein—contains all the amino acids necessary for protein metabolism

complex carbohydrate—a polysaccharide consisting of hundreds or thousands of monosaccharides

consumption norm—the perceived amount of food portion to consume; a form of portion control on food intake

critical period—time during fetal development where the environment has the greatest impact

critical pH—acidic pH of 5.5 where enamel demineralization begins

cruciferous—a family of plants whose leaf structure resemble a cross

crunchy foods—hard dry food that emits sound when chewed

D

defecation—elimination of solid waste

dehydration—abnormal depletion of body fluids

density of bone—thickness of bone mass

detergent foods—foods thought to remove plaque during the action of chewing them

diet—food and drink regularly provided and consumed

dietary guidelines—list of suggestions for healthy eating

dietary supplement—substance that enhances a regular diet

dipeptide—a peptide containing two amino acids

disaccharide—a carbohydrate consisting of two monosaccharide molecules

DRI—abbreviation for dietary reference intake

DRV—British dietary reference value

DV—abbreviation for daily value reported on nutrition labels

dysphagia—difficulty swallowing

E

early childhood caries—syndrome characterized by severe dental caries in teeth of infants and young children

ectomorph—large bone structure

edema—excess accumulation of fluid in body tissues

endomorph—small bone structure

energy balance—an equal amount of energy in (food) and energy out (exercise)

enriched—add nutrients that were lost during food processing

enzymes—proteins that catalyze chemical reactions; assist with breaking apart food molecules during the digestive process

essential amino acids (EAA)—amino acids that must be obtained in the diet

essential fatty acid (EFA)—fatty acid that must be obtained in the diet

essential nutrient—a nutrient the body must get by consuming food

excretion—elimination of toxic waste through body fluids

extracellular—occurring outside a body cell

F

fat soluble—capable of being dissolved in or absorbed by fat

fatty acid—saturated or unsaturated monocarboxylic acids that occur naturally in the form of glycerides in fats and oils

fluoride—compound of fluorine that strengthens tooth enamel and makes it less susceptible to dental caries

food-borne illnesses—sickness that happens due to food laden with bacteria

fortification—adding vitamins and minerals to food products

fruitan—an individual who consumes only raw fruits

functional food—foods or dietary components that may provide a health benefit beyond basic nutrition and impart health benefits or desirable physiological effects

G

gingivitis—inflammation of gingival tissues

glycemic index—rate at which ingested food causes the level of glucose in the blood to rise

goiter—enlargement of the thyroid gland visible from the front of the neck

H

health claims—statements made by food manufacturers that indicate their product will prevent or reduce the risk of certain diseases

heme iron—they type of iron that is readily absorbed by the body; found in animal food products

hemochromatosis—inherited disease where iron builds up in excess in the body

herbal supplement—natural substance thought to heal or improve the human condition

high-density lipoprotein (HDL)—lipoproteins that carry fatty acids and cholesterol from body tissues to the liver

host factors—issues precipitated by the person's own body

hydro—prefix meaning water

hydrogenation—infusing hydrogen at an unsaturated bond between two carbons in a fatty acid to prolong shelf life

homeostasis—stable state of equilibrium

I

immune response—how the body recognizes and defends itself against harmful invading bacteria, viruses, and other detrimental substances

immune system—all the mechanisms within a body that protects against disease by identifying and killing pathogens and tumor cells

incomplete protein—a protein that is missing amino acids to make it complete

inorganic—molecule does not contain carbon

insoluble—does not dissolve in liquid

intracellular—occurring inside a body cell

ionic compound—two or more ions are held next to each other by electrical attraction

K

ketosis—state of metabolism when the liver converts fats to fatty acids and ketones which are then used for energy

kilocalorie—scientific term for calorie

kitchen dangers—anything that might occur in the kitchen that can cause harm to people; fire, illness, injury, and so on

Kwashiorkor—severe malnutrition in infants and children caused by diets that are low in protein

L

lactic acid—most predominant acid formed from bacteria metabolism of carbohydrate

lacto—prefix meaning milk

Lactobacillus—type of oral bacteria responsible for dental caries

lacto-ovo vegetarian—an individual who consumes a vegetarian diet that includes dairy products and eggs

lactovegetarian—an individual who consumes a vegetarian diet that includes dairy products

lanugo—soft, downy growth of hair seen on faces of individuals who starve themselves

lipid—fats and oils

lipoprotein—spherical particles that contain cholesterol, fat, and protein that circulate in the blood

low carb—proportion of carbohydrate in a food product is low compared to protein and fat

low-density lipoprotein (LDL)—lipoprotein that transports cholesterol and triglycerides from the liver to peripheral tissues

lysis—suffix meaning split apart

M

magnesium—fourth most abundant mineral in the human body

major mineral—minerals that are required in the amounts of 100 mg or more

marasmus—chronic malnourishment due to a calorie deficient diet

mastication—chewing food

maternal nutrition—the diet a mother follows when she is pregnant

mesomorph—medium bone structure

methylmercury—methyl group bonded to mercury atom and is highly toxic to the human body

mia—modern abbreviation for bulimia nervosa eating disorder

monosaccharide—one molecule of carbohydrate; is the smallest unit and does not break into a lesser unit

monounsaturated—fatty acid that has a single double bond in the fatty acid chain

mucositis—painful inflammation and ulceration of mucous membranes

MyPyramid—the US government's pictorial graphic that can be individually customized to teach healthy eating habits

N

negative nitrogen balance—nitrogen output exceeds nitrogen intake

neutral pH—7.0 on the pH scale; level at which acid production ceases

NLEA—abbreviation for Nutrition Labeling Education Act of 1990

nonessential amino acids—amino acids made by the body

nonessential nutrient—a nutrient the body produces

nonheme iron—iron that is not well absorbed by the body; found in flour and grains

noxious substance—a substance physically harmful to a human body

nutrition—the sum of the processes by which an animal or plant takes in and utilizes food substances

nutrition facts—name for design of food labels that contain information about a food product

nutrient—a nutritive substance or ingredient

O

oligosaccharide—a carbohydrate containing 3 to 10 monosaccharides

organic—molecule has a carbon-to-carbon bond or carbon-to-hydrogen bond

osmosis—diffusion of fluid through a cell wall

ovo—prefix meaning eggs

P

partially hydrogenated—adding hydrogen to fatty acid to make them more saturated; also called a "trans fat"

peptide—amide derived from two or more amino acids

peptide bond—chemical bond between two molecules formed when a carboxyl group bonds with an amino group

periodontal disease—infection of supporting tissues around teeth

peristalsis—successive waves of involuntary contraction passing along the walls of a hollow muscular structure (as the esophagus or intestine) and forcing the contents onward

phosphate—mineral that helps remineralize enamel

phospholipid—major class of lipid that looks like a triglyceride with a phosphate group

phosphoric acid—ingredient in diet and regular soda that drops the oral pH to acidic levels and contributes to formation of dental caries

plaque biofilm—the layer of micro-organisms that accumulate at the gingival 1/3 in the oral cavity

plaque fluid—solution in and around oral bacterial colonies

polypeptide—chains of amino acids linked by peptide bonds

polyunsaturated—a fatty acid that has two or more double bonds

polysaccharide—a carbohydrate containing many monosaccharide molecules

portion distortion—replacement of proper food consumption norms with larger portions

positive nitrogen balance—nitrogen intake exceeds nitrogen output

posteruptive—period of human development that occurs after teeth are present in the oral cavity

potable—water fit for human consumption

precursor—a biochemical substance from which another more stable substance is formed

pre-eruptive—period of human development before teeth appear in the oral cavity

premature—birth of a child before complete gestation

prenatal—period of development when the child is still a fetus

PRO—abbreviation for protein

purging—to evacuate something unwanted

R

RDA—abbreviation for recommended daily allowance

RDI—abbreviation for recommended daily intake

remineralize—state of repairing demineralized areas of enamel

retentive factor—that which causes food to stick to teeth and not clear the oral cavity readily

roughage—food that contains a lot of fiber

S

safe food handling—practice of keeping, handling, and preparing food so it remains safe for human consumption

saliva—secretion of water, mucin, protein, salts secreted into the mouth by salivary glands

salivary gland hypofunction (SGH)—inadequate saliva production causing dry mouth

satiety—state of feeling full or gratified by food

saturated—having no double or triple bonds between carbons

simple sugar—monosaccharide

SLPI—abbreviation for secretory leukocyte peptidase inhibitor; protective factor in saliva

sodium bicarbonate—baking soda; substance found in saliva that keeps the pH at neutral 7.0

soft foods—food that does not require chewing before swallowing

soluble—able to be dissolved in liquid

solute—a dissolvable substance

starch—category of carbohydrate; plant storage of glucose

sterol—lipids formed with carbon rings instead of chains and fatty acids

Strep mutans—abbreviation for *streptococcus mutans* which is a gram-positive, anaerobic bacteria commonly found in the human oral cavity and is a significant contributor to dental caries

sugar—common name for simple carbohydrate and significant contributor to dental caries

sugar alcohol—hydrogenated form of carbohydrate commonly used for replacing sucrose in food recipes, and does not contribute to tooth decay

supplementary protein—a high quality protein that is added to a meal that is otherwise marginal in protein value

synthesis—combining separate elements to form a whole

synthetic sweetener—noncaloric chemical sweetener that provides sweet taste in a diluted form

T

trace mineral—minerals required in very small amounts

trans fat—fatty acid that has been partially hydrogenated

triglyceride—chemical form in which most fat exists in food as well as in the body

tripeptide—a peptide consisting of three amino acids connected by a peptide bond

V

vegan—an individual who excludes food from their diet that has any animal product in it

very low-density lipoprotein (VLDL)—subclass of lipoprotein that is assembled in the liver from cholesterol and converted in the bloodstream to LDL

W

water soluble—capable of being dissolved in water

X

xylitol—sugar alcohol that is obtained from birch bark, used as a sweetener, and does not contribute to dental caries

Prefixes

mono = one
di= two
tri = three
poly = many
hyper = over
hypo = under
endo = inside
meso = middle
ecto = outside

Suffixes

-ase = enzyme
-ose = carbohydrate
-ine = amino acid

INDEX

Page numbers in *italics* denote figures; numbers with "t" denote table; numbers with "b" indicate box